T0366034

THE FIG
THE MIRACLE FRUIT

FROM ORCHARD
TO BANQUET TABLE

HADI MIRRAFATI

A Special Message to All Athletes

Athletic performance is improved by high carbohydrate diets, not high protein diets. Protein supplements are expensive, unnecessary and even harmful for many people, especially athletes. Athletes need balanced sources of protein and carbohydrates, not concentrated protein. After eating any concentrated protein, like red meat, chicken, fish and milk products, the kidneys must cleanse the blood of protein wastes, such as ammonia, urea, and amino acid fragments. There is a predictable loss of calcium following the ingestion of concentrated protein. For hours after eating a piece of fish or meat, calcium pours out of your body with each urination. This is a well-known and reproducible phenomenon called "protein-induced hypercalcuria" and the calcium that is leaving the blood is being taken out of the body's vital storehouse of calcium—which are the bones. Strong and healthy bones are a very vital component of an athlete's body.

This calcium loss, year after year, drains calcium from the skeleton, resulting in thin, crumbly bones that fracture easily. This is known as osteoporosis. Osteoporosis is most severe in people who consume the most concentrated protein (red meat, chicken, fish, milk and milk products). Fruit and vegetable protein is less prone to cause calcium loss due to its slower absorption and less acidic nature.

Figs are the only fruits that athletes can depend on for protein, carbohydrates, vitamins, minerals and fiber, as well as enzymes. Athletes should definitely avoid fried foods, high-fat meals, lunchmeats, bacon, ham, chicken, fish, milkshakes, and any foods that are cooked in animal fats. Muscles need glycogen (a carbohydrate) for their fuel and carbohydrates give them the sustained energy they need for athletic activity. A basic complex-carbohydrate diet provides sustained, long-term energy. Proteins build tissue and fats provide lubrication and tissue support. Fiber allows good elimination. Female athletes need iron-rich foods, as their red blood cells may be broken down more rapidly. Figs do all of these as well as provide vitamins, minerals and salts.

Athletes: stay away from alcohol, cigarette smoking, coffee, black tea and cola beverages. Your best herb teas are green tea, ginseng tea, comfrey tea and white willow bark tea. For enhanced taste, use dried figs with your tea. Eat a few dried figs with a cup of green tea before you exercise, train or compete.

To my sons

Kamran and Kamfar

ISBN: Softcover 978-1-4134-5465-9
Hardcover 978-1-4134-5466-6
EBook 979-8-3694-1978-6

To order additional copies of this book, contact:
Xlibris
844-714-8691
www.Xlibris.com
Orders@Xlibris.com

Print information available on the last page

Rev. date: 04/10/2024

Contents

Chapter One

NATURE'S MIRACLE FRUIT

There is something magical about fruit trees that bear beautiful flowers and edible fruit. An edible fruit that contains the nutrients we need - vitamins, minerals, enzymes, fibers, protein, carbohydrates and fat- is a miracle of nature. It is our duty to introduce fruit trees and their benefits to our new generation. We need to protect these trees and supply them with healthy conditions. Our purpose is to encourage more growers to invest in the cultivation and production of orchards planted with the miracle fruit: the fig.

The Ficus carica of the Moraceae family is known familiarly as figue (French), feige (German), figo (Italian), higo or brevo(Spanish) and fig (English). Figs are not technically fruits in the botanical sense; they are hundreds of minuscule flowers encased in fleshy balloon-like receptacles (syconium) that we conveniently term fruit. Figs contain fiber and minerals that are medically curative and dietetically delicious: **They can "clean inside" and help create a "youthful outside."**

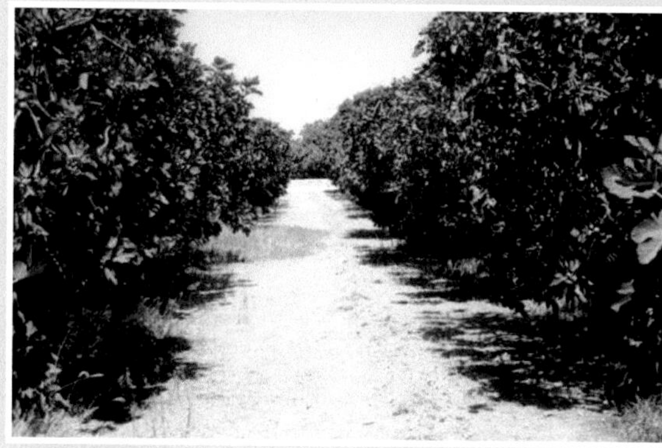

A Fig Orchard

Today, we know that the fig is a significant source of fiber, which helps prevent colon cancer. More fiber in your diet also lowers cholesterol and thus the risk of heart disease. Three figs, dried or fresh, provide about 5 grams of fiber, 20 percent of your daily requirement. That amount can go a long way. Figs are particularly good for people who are overweight, another risk for heart disease. They stay in the stomach longer, therefore, helping people eat less. They are also very sweet, satisfying those cravings.

Figs can be an important orchard crop for growers who want to invest in a crop with universal appeal to good taste and health benefits you can bring to market.

General Description

The adult fig tree ranges from 10 to 30 feet high, with numerous spreading branches and a trunk rarely more than seven inches in diameter, which contains milky latex. The root system is typically shallow and spreading, sometimes covering fifty feet of ground. Fig wood is weak and decays rapidly. The trunk often bears large nodule tumors, where branches have been shed or removed. The twigs are cylindrical and pithy rather than woody. The deciduous leaves are palmate, deeply divided into three to seven main lobes.

Fig leaves are bright green, single, alternate and large (to one foot length). They are rough and hairy on the upper surface and soft and hairy on the underside. The fruit is a fleshy, hollow receptacle with a small opening at the apex partly closed by small scales. It may be obovoid, rather oval shaped with the narrow end at the base, turbinate or pear shaped, one to four inches long. It varies in color from yellowish-green to coppery-bronze or dark-purple. Tiny flowers are massed on the inside wall and out of sight, clustered inside the green "fruit." Common fig flowers are all female and need no pollination. Smyrna figs require pollination by a fig wasp, Blastophaga psenes. Figs that require wasp-pollination consist of two groups of trees, the caprifig and the edible fig. The caprifig produces an inedible false-fruit that is the habitat for the wasp. Caprifigs are picked just before the wasps emerge and are hung in the trees of the edible figs. The San Pedro fig needs pollination for its second and succeeding crops. The skin of the fig is thin and tender. Its fleshy wall is whitish, pale-yellow, amber or more or less pink, rose, red or purple. The fig is juicy and sweet when ripe, but gummy with latex when unripe. Its seeds are medium or small and range in number from 30 to 1,600 per fruit. Figs have one of the shortest life-spans of any fruit.

Origin and Distribution

The fig has been cultivated for centuries in warm, semi-arid climates. The fig is believed to be indigenous to western Asia and to have been distributed by man throughout the Mediterranean area. Figs were also part of the athlete's diet for the original Olympic games in ancient Greece. Because they give you a great energy boost during the day, we can call them the **athlete's fruit!**

Fig growing territory gradually stretched from Afghanistan to southern Germany and the Canary Islands. Figs were introduced into England in the sixteenth century. By 1550 they were reported to be in Chinese gardens. European types were taken to China, Japan, India, South Africa, and Australia. When the Spanish set out to the New World in the 1500's they brought figs to Mexico, planted along such staple crops as grapevines and sugarcane in their new colonies. Thomas Jefferson was another contributor to the spread of the fig trees throughout the southern United States. He brought three different varieties of fig home from France. A century ago figs were still a major crop

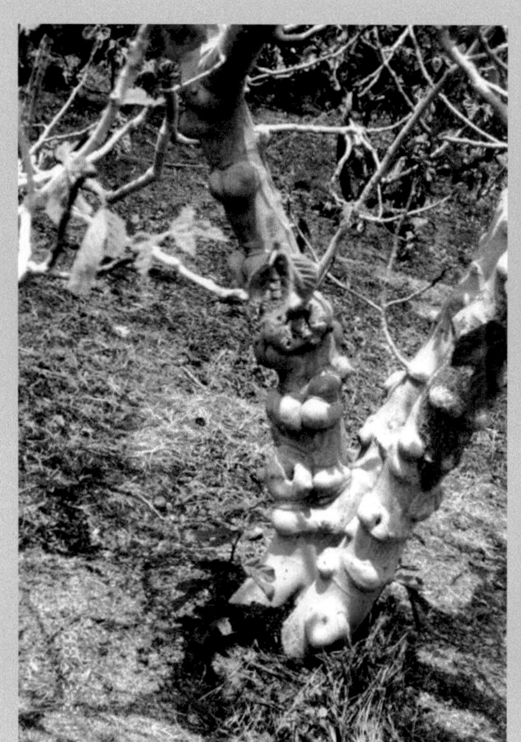

A Fig Orchard

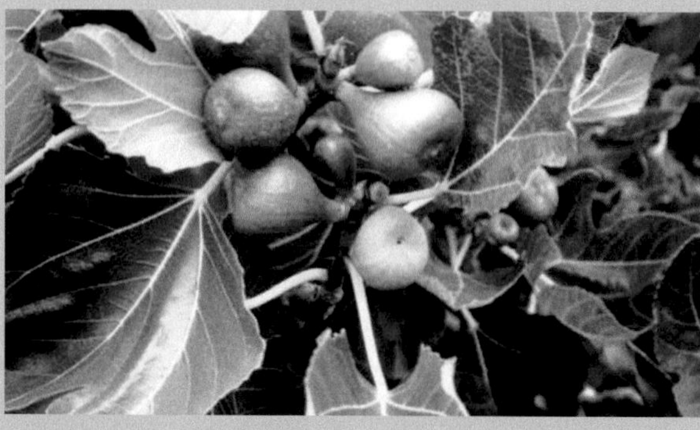

Late Spring Fig Tree Fruits

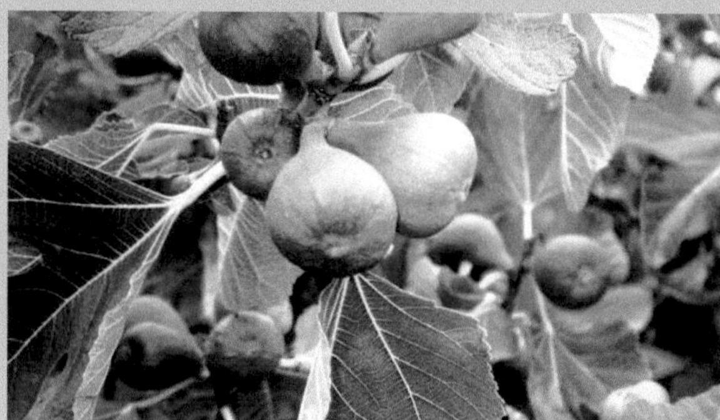

Summer Figs

in Florida, Virginia, and other southern states. Times and tastes changed and commercial production stopped, but the fig has remained on the table and in the landscape. Turkish varieties are still a common sight in Florida, Georgia, Louisiana, Virginia, South Carolina, Tennessee and Mississippi. In California, figs were introduced when the San Diego Mission was established in 1769.

The fig tree was planted in Bermuda in colonial times and was common around Bahamian plantations. It became a familiar dooryard plant in the West Indies and at medium and low altitude in Central America and Northern South America. There are fair-sized plantations on mountain sides of Honduras, at low elevations on the Pacific side of Costa Rica, from Florida to northern South America, to Chile and Argentina where cooler zoned types are grown.

Climate or Adaptation

The fig grows best and produces the best quality fruit in Mediterranean and dryer warm-temperature climates. Rains during fruit development and ripening can cause the fruit to split. With extra care, figs will also grow in wetter, cooler areas. Fully dormant trees can remain hardy in 12 to 15 degrees F, but plants in active growth can be damaged at 30 degrees F. Only the hardiest cultivars (plants that are cultivated, rather than naturally growing) can be grown in areas such as the Willamette Valley, the Sierra Nevada, and the high desert. All cultivars are suitable elsewhere in California. Chilling requirements for the fig are less than 300 hours. It is best to choose a slow-growing cultivar. In tropical areas generally, figs thrive between altitudes of 2,600 and 5,900 feet. The tree can tolerate 10 to 20 degrees of frost in favorable sites, but it should have dry climate with light early spring rains if the production of fresh fruit is desired. The semiarid tropical and subtropical regions of the world are ideal, if irrigation is available, making California an excellent location for cultivation. Very hot, dry spells cause fruit-drop, even if the trees are irrigated. Figs require full sun all day to ripen palatable fruits. The fig tree becomes enormous and will shade out anything growing beneath. The succulent trunk and branches are unusually sensitive to heat and sun damage, and should be whitewashed if particularly exposed. The roots are greedy, traveling far beyond the tree canopy; therefore, the fig tree is not for small places.

Soil

The fig can be grown on a wide range of soils: light sand, rich loam, heavy clay and limestone, with sufficient depth and good drainage. Sandy, medium dry soil that contains a good deal of lime is preferred when the crop is intended for drying. Highly acidic soil is unsuitable and the pH should be between 6.0 and 6.5. The tree is fairly tolerant of moderate salinity.

Propagation

Fig plants are usually propagated by cutting foot-long pieces of dormant wood, less than one inch in diameter, with two-year-old wood at base. Dip the cuttings in a rooting hormone and allow them to callus one week in a moist place at 50 to 60 degrees F. Summer cuttings may also be made, but they do best if defoliated and winterized in refrigeration for two to three weeks before potting. Leafy shoots require a mist bed. Cultivars may be propagated on rootstocks or older trees, top worked by whip, cleft or crown grafting or chip or patch buildings. Rooted cuttings should be planted in areas of 22 to 30 square feet, depending upon the capacity of the soil and the ultimate size of the tree. Keep the roots moist until planted. Never transplant or disturb a young tree while it is starting new growth in spring. Cut the tree back to two feet in length upon planting and whitewashing the trunk. Trees have been raised from seeds and even seeds extracted in air layering can be planted satisfactorily. There is rapid mass multiplication by tissue. Size of the cutting should be half-to three-quarters of an inch in thickness and eight to twelve inches in length.

Harvesting the Dried Crop

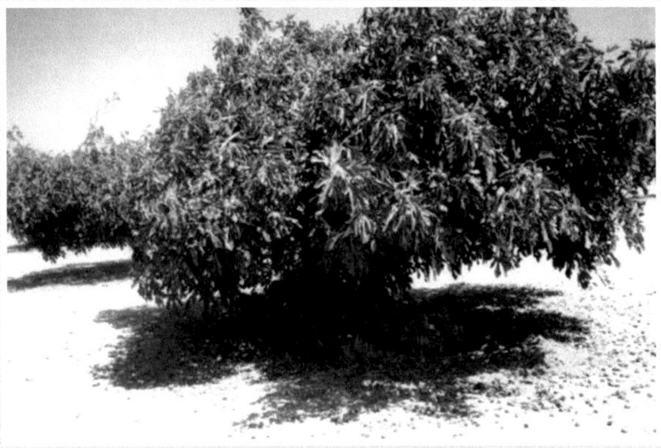

Irrigation

Young fig trees should be watered regularly until fully established. In dry western climate, mature trees should be watered deeply at least every one or two weeks. Desert gardeners may have to water more frequently. Mulch the soil around the trees to conserve moisture. If a tree is not getting enough water, the leaves will turn yellow and drop. Drought-stressed trees will not produce fruit and are more susceptible to nematode damage.

Harvesting

Fig cultivation may produce one to two crops per year. Small amounts of hand-picked figs are marketed fresh. Most figs are harvested as a dried crop: allowed to dry on the tree and fall to the ground. Dried figs are mechanically swept into windrows and collected. Harvest is repeated at two-to three-week intervals. The figs are fumigated, sun-dried or dehydrated to 17 percent moisture or less. The fruit may be picked from the tree or gathered by mechanical sweepers after they fall to the ground. Some figs are so tender they must be picked when slightly unripe in order to be firm enough for processing. Workers must wear gloves and protective clothing because of the latex. Harvested fruit are spread out in the shade for a day so that the latex will dry a little, then they are transported to processing plants in wooden boxes.

Harvested Fruit

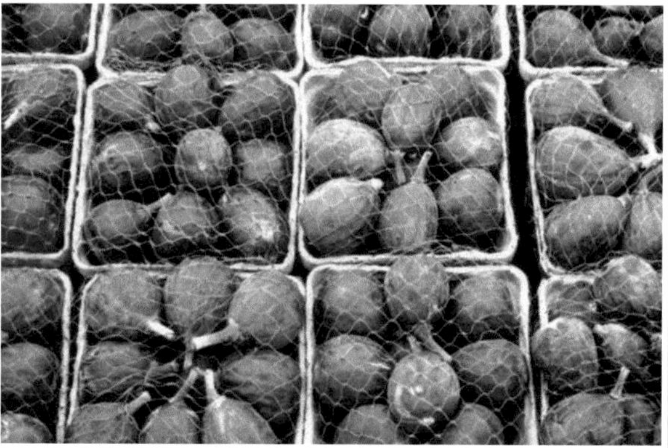

Pruning

Fig trees grow quite rapidly to a height between 15 and 30 feet. They are typically low branched and spreading. These fruiters are grown on their roots and can live for 100 years or more. Where hard freezes are common, the wood freeze back severely and the plant turns into a big shrub. In some colder areas, the plants will dry to the ground each winter, but will send up new shoots in spring. Under the most favorable growing conditions most fig varieties produce two crops a year. The first is in early summer from wood formed the previous year. The second appears in late summer, borne at the ends of new growth that formed while the first crop of figs was maturing. In colder climates only the second crop is produced, while in cool summer areas only the first crop ripens. A fig is somewhat indifferent to pruning because it can take quite a bit, yet still bear an ample crop. It will also bear without pruning.

In climates where the plant freezes, any pruning consists mainly of removing damaged stems after growth resumes in the spring. Dried, weak or crossing branches should be pruned. Fig trees are produced with or without heavy pruning; however, it is essential to prune only during the initial years. Trees should be trained according to use of fruit (low crown for fresh market figs). Once the tree form is established, the crop is borne on the terminal of previous year's wood. Heavy winter pruning should be avoided. This causes loss of the following year's crop. It is better to prune immediately after the main crop is harvested. In summer, prune half the branches and prune the remainder the following summer. If radical pruning is done, whitewash the entire tree. To increase the harvest, train the tree to an open center, keeping the main scaffold limbs close to the ground. After a main framework has formed, prune to encourage new wood and to remove crowded stems in the center. Do any major pruning during the dormant season. However, with two crops, avoid cutting back heavily between them as it can seriously reduce the size of the second crop and remove growth that will carry the next year's first crop.

FERTILIZATION

Regular fertilizing of figs is usually necessary only for potted trees or when they are grown on sands. Excess nitrogen encourages rank growth at the expense of fruit production and the fruit produced often ripens improperly, if at all. Generally, fig trees should be fertilized if the branches grow less than a foot from the previous year. Apply about 1 pound of actual nitrogen divided into three or four applications beginning in late winter or early spring and ending in July.

PESTS AND DISEASES

PESTS

Fig tree roots are a favorite food of gophers which can easily kill a large plant. One passive method of control is to plant the tree in a large aviary wire basket. Birds can cause a lot of damage to the fruit. Fig trees are prone to attack by nematodes, particularly in sandy soils, where they attack the roots, forming galls and stunting the trees. Driedfruit beetles of the *Nitidulidae* family have a wide host range and will infest any ripe fruit. *Carpophilus hemipterus* is the most common species, but the Freeman sap beetle and the Confused sap beetle (*c. freemani* and *c. mutilatus* are also common. Beetles enter ripening fruit through the eye and cause damage by introducing fungi and knots. They are especially harmful to Calimyrna which have a large eye and is easily infested. Euryphid mites cause little damage, but are carriers of Fig Mosaic virus from infected trees

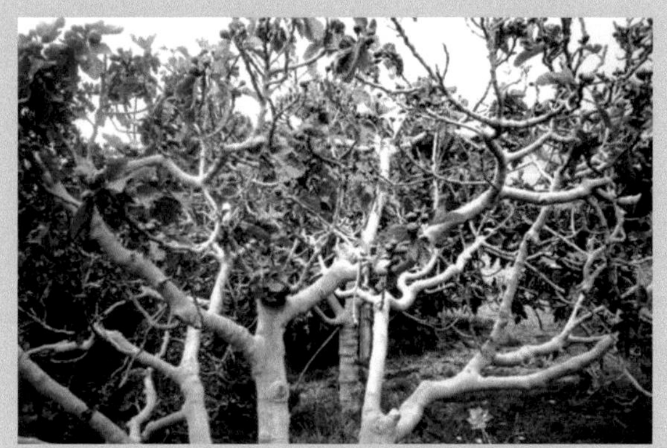

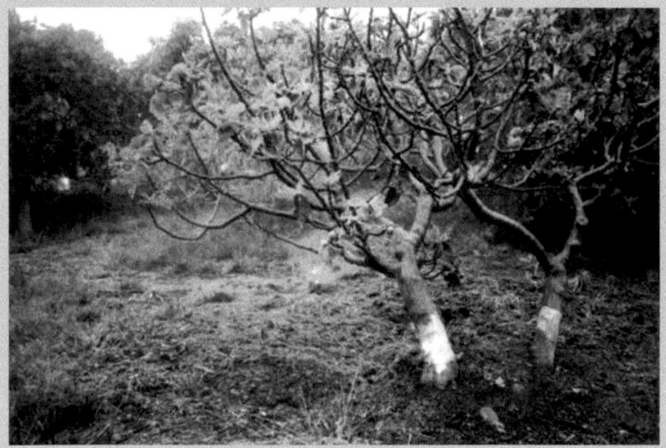

Spring Time Fig Trees

to clean trees. Batocera stem-boring beetles feed on branches and may kill the tree. Lepidosaphes conchiformis scale feed on leaves, twigs and fruit. The larvae of the fig borer *Azochis Gripusali* feed on the new growth, tunnel down through the trees to the roots and kill the tree. Epitrix and Colaspis beetles perforate and severely damage the leaves and shoots. Sucking insects called *Asterolecanium* attack the bark.

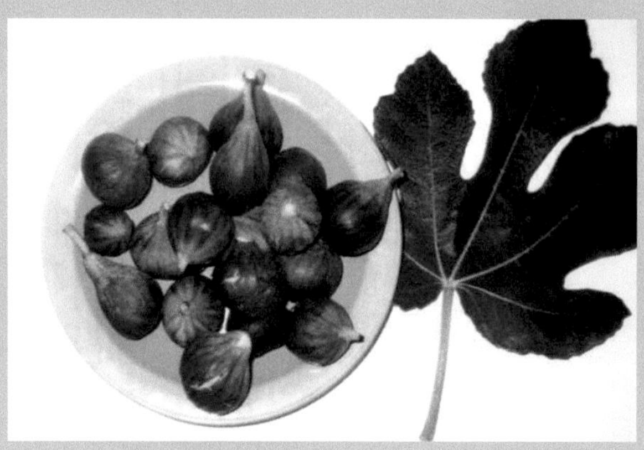

Magnolia Fig

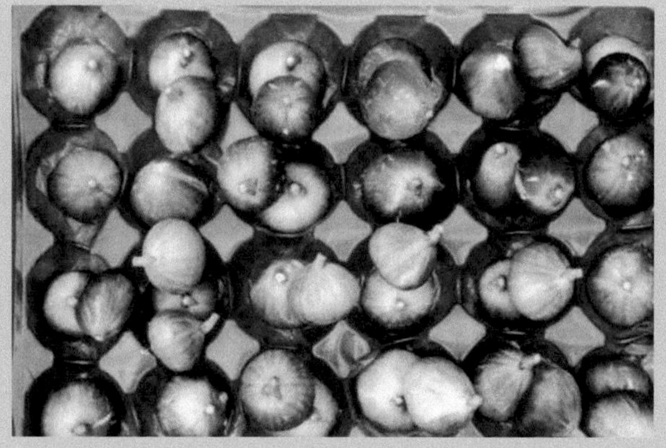

Celeste or Honey Fig

DISEASES

A common and widespread problem is leaf rust caused by Veroteluim Fici, which causes premature leaf fall and reduces yields. Leaf spot results from infection by *Clindrocladium Scoparium* or *Cerospora Fici*. Fig Mosaic is caused by a virus, and results in leaves that are marbled with yellow spots and light colored veins. *Botrytes* causes a blast of branch terminals which dry out and turn charcoal-like. Fig canker is a bacterium which enters the trunk at damage zones, causing necrosis and girdling and loss of branches. Rhyzopus smut attacks ripened fruit on the tree, causing charcoal black coating inside the fruit. Fig Endosepsis caused by *fusaruim moniliforme* or *fusarium solani* is a disease carried by the Fig Wasp and affects the fruit of those varieties that are pollinated by the wasp. *Aspergillus* fungus rots the fruit and appears to burst or as a ropy mucous-like exudates drums from the eye. Penicillium fungus will attack dried fruit in storage.

VARIETIES

There are many cultivated varieties of figs. The characteristics we describe may help you choose those best suited for your area.

- **Celeste (Blue Celeste, Honey Fig, Malta, Sugar, Violette)**
  - Best in temperate climate
  - Pear-shaped
  - Ribbed
  - Short neck and slender stalk to ¾ inch long
  - The eye (opening at apex) is closed
  - The fruit is small to medium

- The skin is purplish-brown or bronze tinged with purple
- The pulp is whitish or pinkish amber
- Rich flavor, good quality and sweet
- Almost seedless
- Main crop is heavy but of short duration
- Productive
- Hardy
- Usually dried

- **Brown Turkey (Aubiquc, Noire, Negro Largo, San Piero)**
  - Broad-pyriform
  - Usually without neck
  - Medium to large
  - Copper-colored
  - Pulp is whitish shading to pink or light red
  - Good to very good quality
  - With few seeds
  - Best when fresh
  - Hardy
  - The tree is prolific and vigorous
  - The main crop begins in mid-July and is large
  - Adopted to warm climates
  - Does best in Southern California

- **Brunswick (Magnolia)**
  - Leaves narrow-lobed
  - Fruit of main crop are oblique-turbinate
  - Mostly without neck
  - Fruit stalk thick
  - Often swollen
  - Fruit of medium size
  - Bronze or purplish-brown
  - Pulp whitish near skin, shading to pink or amber, hollow in center
  - Fair to good quality
  - Nearly seedless
  - Ripen over a long season
  - Breba crop poor, large, bronze-skinned, flesh light-red

- **Marseilles (Blanche, Italian Honey Fig, Lattarula, Lemon Fig, White Marseilles)**
  - Fruit of main crop round to oblate without neck
  - Slender stalks to ¼ inch long
  - Medium size
  - Very sweet
  - Lemon flavor
  - Breba crop with turbinate with short, thick neck and short stalk
  - Skin yellow green
  - Flesh white to amber
  - Seed large and conspicuous
  - Fair quality

- **Adriatic (Fragola, Strawberry Fig, Verdone, White Adriatic)**
  - All-purpose fig
  - Small to medium
  - Skin greenish
  - Flesh strawberry colored

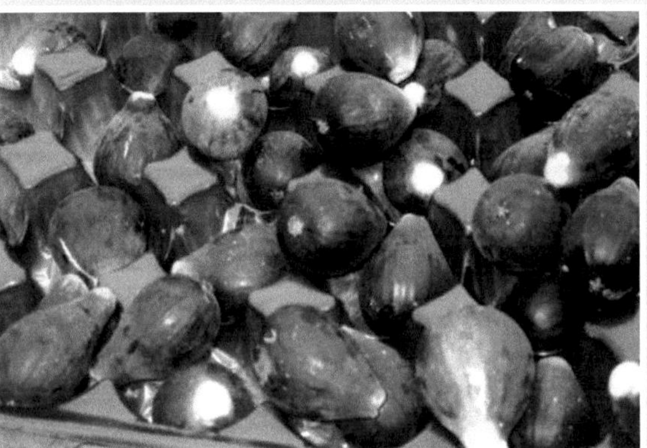

Mission Fig

- Good and very good quality
- All purpose fig
- Turbinate with short, thick neck and short stalk
- Light breba crop with fruit oblique-pyriform
- Subject to frost damage
- Prune to force new growth

- **Genoa (White Genoa)**
  - Pyriform or turbinate
  - Very faintly ribbed
  - Neck thick and short or absent
  - Medium size
  - Skin downy, greenish-yellow to white
  - Flesh yellow-amber near skin, mostly amber tinged with red
  - Sweet, good for fresh or dried
  - Fruit of breba crop oblique-obovate with thick neck and short stalk
  - Tree upright
  - Requires constant annual pruning
  - Best adopted to cooler regions of the west

- **Purple Genoa (Black Genoa, Black Spanish)**
  - Oblong, broad at apex, narrow at base
  - Large size
  - Very dark-purple with thick blue bloom
  - Pulp yellowish becoming reddish to red the center
  - Juicy
  - Sweet with rich flavor

- **Black Ischia (Blue Ischia)**
  - Main crop is elongated pear shaped
  - Short neck and short to medium stalk
  - Dark purple-black except at the apex where it is lighter and greenish with many golden flecks
  - Skin is fully coated with thin, dark blue bloom
  - Eye open with red-violet scales
  - Pulp is violet-red
  - Good quality
  - In their breba crop, the fruit is small and pulp is red
  - The tree is particularly ornamental and leaves are glossy

- **Peona**
  - Bell shaped
  - Medium size
  - Thin skinned
  - Light purple with red flesh
  - Sweet
  - Good flavor

- **Black Mission (Bears Black, Franciscan)**
  - Fruits all over black-purple
  - Elongated

Dried Mission Figs

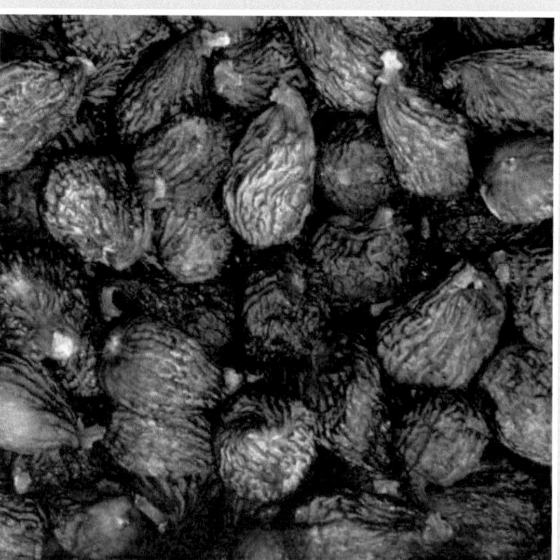

- Flesh watermelon to pink
- Fairly good taste
- Easily dried at home
- Single best all round variety for south, north coast
- Brebas prolific, fairly rich
- Tree very large
- Interior location

- **Conadria**
  - Fruit pale green
  - Medium size
  - Flesh strawberry-red
  - Mildly sweet
  - Good fresh
  - Excellent dried
  - Light breba crop
  - Best in hot climates

- **Croisic (Cordelia, Gillette, St. John Fig)**
  - Only edible Capri fig
  - Fruit very early
  - Fruits pale yellow
  - Small size
  - Pulp nearly white
  - Tree low, dense spreading
  - For north coast and pacific northwest

- **Desert King (Charlie, King Fig)**
  - Large size
  - Skin is deep green, minutely spotted white
  - Pulp strawberry-red
  - Sweet
  - Delicious fresh or dried
  - Tree highly vigorous
  - Hardy
  - Best adapted to cool area, Pacific northwest

- **Excel**
  - Large size
  - Skin is yellow
  - Flesh light amber
  - Fruits practically neck-less
  - Very sweet
  - Excellent all purpose fig
  - Light breba crop
  - More productive

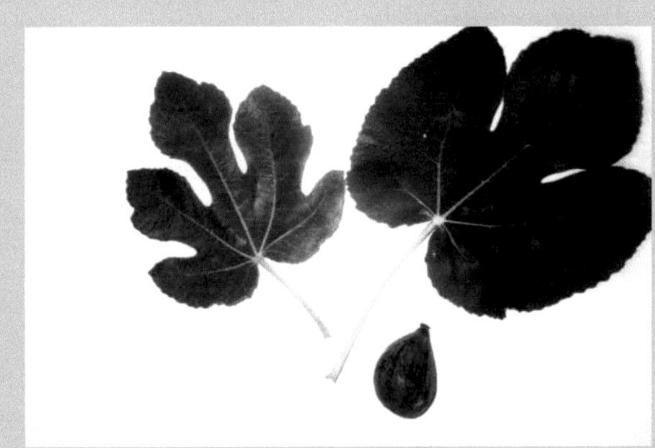

Black Mission Fig and Leaf

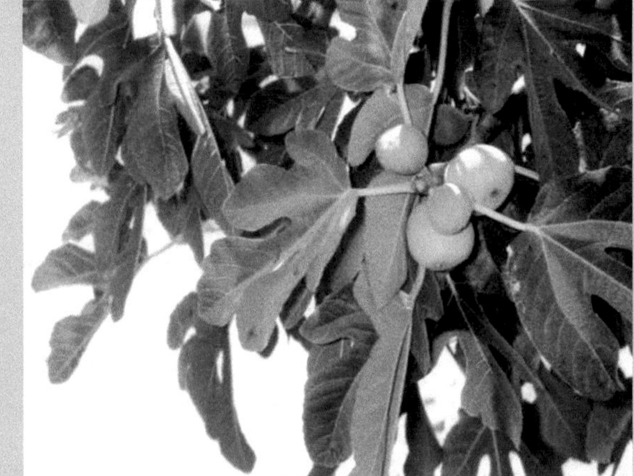

Calimyrna Fig

- Tree vigorous
- Does well in most parts of California

- **Flanders**
  - Medium size
  - Long neck
  - Skin is brownish-yellow with violet stripes
  - Flesh amber
  - Strong, fine flavor
  - Excellent all purpose fruit
  - Good breba crop
  - Ripens late
  - Tree vigorous
  - For south coastal California, San Joaquin Valley

- **Kadota (Dottato, Florentine, White Kadota)**
  - Medium size
  - Skin yellowish-green
  - Flesh amber, tinged pink at center
  - Flavor rich
  - Resists souring
  - Little or no breba crop
  - Tree upright
  - Requires hot, dry climate for best quality

Fresh Calimyrna Fig

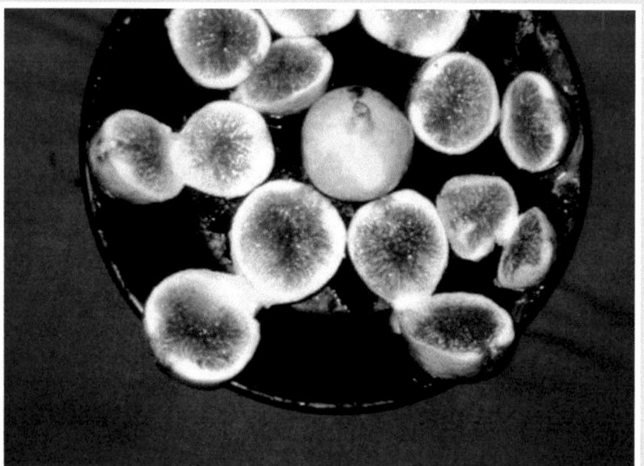

- **Osborn's Prolific (Arachipel, Neveralla)**
  - Medium to large
  - Skin is dark, reddish-brown
  - Flesh amber, often tinged pink
  - Very sweet
  - Best fresh
  - Light breba crop
  - Tree upright, bare
  - Will grow in shade
  - Ripens late
  - Only for north coast, Pacific northwest
  - Poor in warm climate

- **Panachee (Stripped Tiger, Tiger)**
  - Small to medium
  - Skin is greenish-yellow with dark green stripes
  - Flesh strawberry
  - Sweet
  - Best fresh
  - No breba crop
  - Requires long, warm growing season
  - Ripens late

- **Tena**
  - Small size
  - Light green skin
  - Flesh amber
  - Fine flavor
  - Good fresh or dried
  - Good breba crop
  - Bears heavily
  - Tree strong, dense
  - For coastal California
  - Interior south

- **Ventura**
  - Large size
  - Green skin
  - Deep red flesh

- Long neck
  - Excellent flavor
  - Good fresh or dried
  - Good breba crop
  - Ripens late
  - Compact tree

- **Vente (Green Ischia)**
  - Small size
  - Greenish-yellow skin
  - Flesh strawberry
  - Excellent fresh or dried
  - Good breba crop
  - Small tree
  - For short summer climates

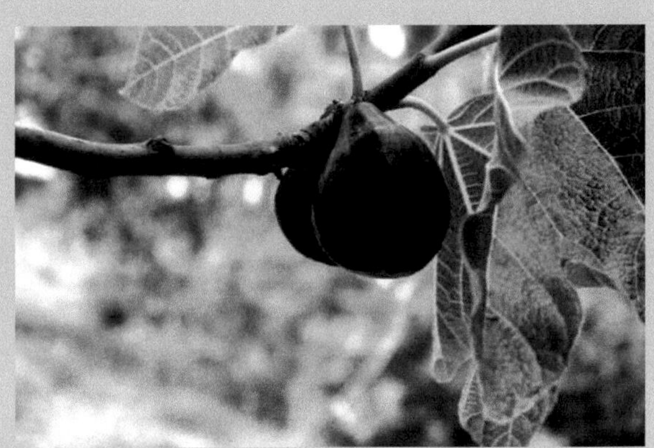

Mission Fig on Branch

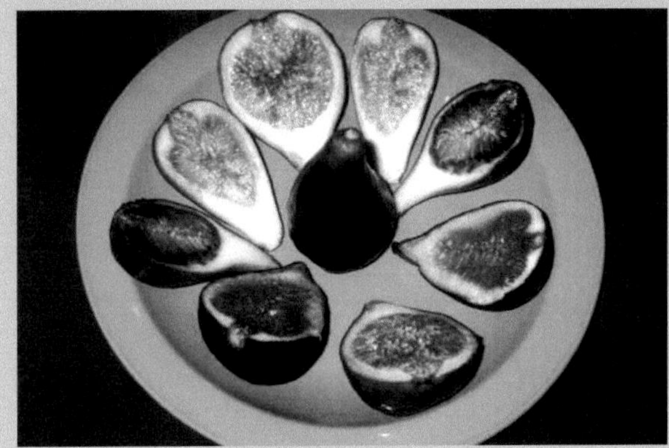

Fresh Figs

STORAGE

Fresh market figs must be harvested when almost fully ripe to be of best eating quality. A fresh fig's skin color and flesh firmness is related to its quality and post harvest-life.

Recommendations for maintaining post harvest quality are given here.

- Maturity Indices:
  - Skin color and flesh firmness are dependable maturity and ripeness indices.
  - Black Mission figs should be light to dark purple than black and should yield to slight pressure.
  - Calimyrna figs should be yellowish-white to light and firm.
- Quality Indices:
  - Flavor is influenced by stage of ripeness.
  - Over ripe figs can become undesirable due to fermentative products.
  - Other quality indices include insects and decay, and absence of defects, such as bind-peck, sunburn, scab, skin break, and stem shrivel.
- Optimum Temperature:
  - 30 to 32 degrees F.
  - Expedited forced-air cooling to 32 degrees F is strongly recommended.
  - Optimum relative humidity is 90-95 percent.

- To calculate heat production, multiply ml CO2/Kg.Hr. by 440 to get B/ton/day or by 122 to get Kcal/metric ton/day (Table 1).

Table 1. Rate of Respiration Production

Temperature		Production
F	C	ml CO_2/Kg.Hr
32	0	2-4
41	5	5-8
50	10	9-12
68	20	20-30

- Rates of Ethylene Production:

Temperature		Production
F	C	C2H4/KgHr
32	0	0.4-0.8
41	5	0.8-1.5
50	10	1.5-3.0
68	20	4.0-6.0

- Responses to Ethylene:
  - Figs are slightly sensitive to ethylene action on stimulating softening and decay severity, especially if kept at 41° F or higher temperature.
- Responses to controlled atmospheres:
  - Controlled atmospheres of 5-10 percent oxygen and 15-20 percent carbon dioxide are effective in decay control, firmness, retention, and reduction of respiration and ethylene production rates.
  - Post-harvest life at optimum temperature and relative humidity depends upon cultivator and ripeness stage at harvest and ranges from one to two weeks in air, and from three to four weeks in controlled atmospheres for California-grown Black Mission and Calimyrna Figs.
- Physiological and Physical Disorders:
  - Controlled atmospheres - relative disorders
  - Extended storage in controlled atmospheres can result in loss of characteristic flavors.
  - Figs exposed to less than 2 percent oxygen and or more than 25 percent carbon dioxide develop off-flavor due to fermentative metabolism.
- Pathological Disorders:
  - Alternaria tenuis or Alternario rot appears as small, round, brown-to-black spots over the fruit surface.
  - Any cracks on the skin make the fruit more susceptible to rot.
  - *Aspergillus niger* or black mold rot. Appears as dark or yellowish spots in the flesh with no external symptoms.
  - At advanced stages the skin and flesh turn slightly pink color and white mycelia and black spore masses follow.
  - *Fusarium moniliforme* or soft rot appears in the cavity of the fig making the pulp soft, watery and brown with sometimes an offensive odor. Souring is a pre-harvest problem resulting from yeast and bacteria carried into the figs by insects, especially vinegar flies, resulting in smells of alcohol or acetic acid.
- Keeping Quality:
  - Fresh figs are very perishable.
  - At 40° F to 43° F and 75 percent relative humidity, figs remain in good condition

for eight days, but have a shelf life of only one to two days when removed from storage.

- At 50° F and relative humidity of 85 percent, figs can be kept no longer than 21 days.
- They remain in good condition for 30 days when stored at 32° F to 35° F
- If frozen whole, they can be maintained for several months.

Leaves

Fig leaves plucked after the fruit harvest are sometimes used for fodder. In France, and some other countries, there is some use of fig leaves as a source of perfume material called "Fig-leaf absolute."

Latex and Other Uses

Latex contains caoutichouc (pure rubber), resin, albumin, cerin, sugar, malic acid, renrin, proteolytic enzymes, diastase, esterase, lipase, cutalase, peroxidase. It is collected at its peak of activity in early morning, then dried and powdered for use in coagulating milk to make cheese and junket. From it can be isolated the protein-digesting enzyme ficin, which is used for tenderizing meat, rendering fat, and clarifying beverages. Usually, the fruits are allowed to ripen fully and partially dehydrate on the tree, then are exposed to sulphur fumes for about one half hour. They are placed in the sun and turned daily to achieve uniform drying. Some longer varieties are pressed flat during the five-to seven-day process. Black Mission and Kadota figs are suitable for freezing whole in syrup or sliced and layered with sugar. Dried cull figs have been roasted and ground as a coffee substitute. In some countries, low-grade figs are converted into alcohol. An alcoholic extract of dried figs has been used as a flavor for liqueurs and tobacco. Figs can supply seed oil. Dried seeds contain 30 percent of a fixed oil containing fatty acids. Its edible oil can also be used as a lubricant.

We hope you are interested in the fig as an orchard crop, whose leaves, seed and fruit offer many products for today's markets.

Chapter Two

GROWING AND PRODUCING FIGS

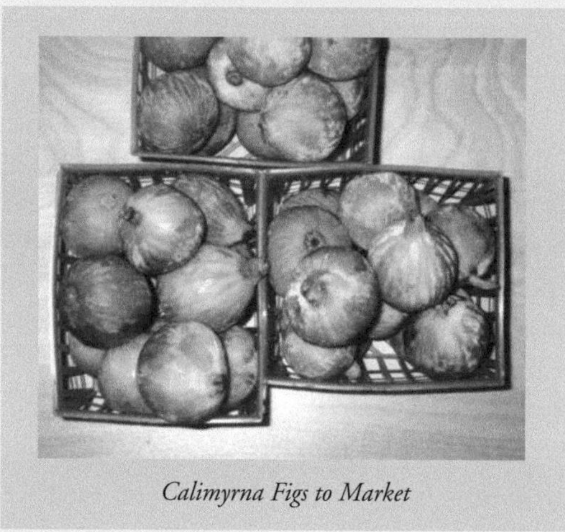

Calimyrna Figs to Market

Perhaps now you are ready to begin growing and producing figs to feed a healthy nation and world appetite. How do you go about it? What will be the costs and what will be your return on your investment? What factors do you have to consider in the way of equipment, labor, irrigation, acreage and cultivation practices?

To help you begin growing and producing a fig crop or improve on the orchard you may now have, we consulted the University of California at Davis, one of the most prominent centers for the study of agri-business, especially related to our subject, the fig. In 1994, the UC Davis Cooperative Extension conducted a comprehensive study of fig production in California's San Joaquin Valley. Because of its intricate breakdown of a fig grower's operation, it serves as an excellent model for growers today, even years later. With kind permission from UC Davis, we re-print the Calimyrna study in full, including Tables, and the text only of the Black Mission and Conadria Fig studies. The Tables for these studies are not included but can be found on the

Cooperative Extension website, below. Some of the costs in these studies have changed over the years. UC Cooperative Extension suggests that our readers consult the Cooperative Extension and Outreach departments of the Land Grant College or University in their geographic area for more recent information on costs and yields. You can find a list of the Land Grant schools on the website www.nasulgc.org/publications/Land_Grant/Schools.htm. Because fig production is stable in the U.S., more recent studies on fig production have not been performed. The reader can find studies on related crops, such as almonds, prunes, raisins and wine grapes for information. The UC Davis Cooperative Extension runs production costs and returns studies on an annual basis. Links to these studies can be located on their website http://fruitsandnuts/ucdavis.edu. There you will also find the complete costs and yields studies for the Black Mission and Conadria fig studies, including the tables. Growers in southern states, such as Georgia, Florida, Louisiana, Alabama and Mississippi will find help from their cooperative extensions through a web link www.growinglifestyle.com. The California Fig Advisory Board also has information that will help you at www.californiafigs.com.

U.C. COOPERATIVE EXTENSION

GENERAL INFORMATION
FOR ESTABLISHING A FIG ORCHARD AND PRODUCING FIGS
Calimyrna Variety - San Joaquin Valley - 1994

The detailed costs for establishment and production of the Calimyrna variety of figs in the San Joaquin Valley are presented in this study. The hypothetical farm used in this report consists of 500 acres, all of which are in fig production.

Practices described in this study are based on those production procedures considered typical for this crop and area. Additional practices not listed may be required. Sample costs given for labor, materials, equipment and contract services are based on current figures. Some costs and practices detailed in this study may not be applicable to your situation. This study is only intended as a guide and can be used in making production decisions, determining potential returns, preparing budgets, and evaluating production loans. A blank Your Cost column is provided to enter your actual costs on **Table 2, Sample Costs to Produce Figs and Table 3, Costs and Returns Per Acre To Produce Figs.**

This study consists of General Assumptions For Establishing A Fig Orchard And Producing Figs and seven tables. Tables included:

Table 1. Costs Per Acre to Establish A Fig Orchard
Table 2. Costs Per Acre to Produce Figs
Table 3. Costs and Returns Per Acre To Produce Figs
Table 4. Monthly Cash Costs Per Acre to Produce Figs
Table 5. Whole Farm Annual Equipment, Investment and Business Overhead Costs
Table 6. Hourly Equipment Costs
Table 7. Ranging Analysis

For an explanation of calculations used for the study refer to the attached General Assumptions or call the Department of Agricultural Economics, Cooperative Extension, University of California, Davis, California, (530) 752-3563 or call the farm advisor in the county of interest.

Two additional cost of production studies for different varieties of figs grown in this region are also available: "Sample Costs To Establish A Fig Orchard And Produce Figs, Conadria Variety In the San Joaquin Valley - 1994" and "Sample Costs to Establish A Fig Orchard And Produce Figs, Black Mission Variety In the San Joaquin Valley - 1994."

The studies mentioned above can be requested through the Department of Agricultural Economics, U.C. Davis or from selected county Cooperative Extension offices.

GENERAL ASSUMPTIONS
FOR ESTABLISHING A FIG ORCHARD AND PRODUCING FIGS
Calimyrna Variety - San Joaquin Valley - 1994

The following contains some general assumptions pertaining to sample costs of Calimyrna variety fig orchard establishment and production in the San Joaquin Valley. Practices described should not be considered recommendations by the University of California, but rather represent production procedures considered typical for this crop and area. Some of these costs and practices may not be applicable to a specific situation nor used during every production year. Additional ones not indicated may be needed. Establishment and cultural practices for the production of figs vary by grower and region. Variations can be significant. The practices and inputs used in this cost study serve only as a sample or guide. These costs are represented on an annual, per acre basis. *The use of trade names in this report does not constitute an endorsement or recommendation by the University of California nor is any criticism implied by omission of other similar products.*

1. <u>LAND:</u>

The farm consists of 500 acres of land. There are 80 acres currently being established in the actual fig orchard with another 415 acres on which figs are grown and 5 acres of roads and farmstead. No other crops are grown. Land is valued at $1,200 per acre and is not depreciated.

2. <u>TREES:</u>

The specific variety of fig trees planted in this study are Calimyrna. The trees are planted at 15 x 20 foot spacing, with 155 trees per acre. Fig trees have a very long production life if they are well maintained. Some fig orchards in the San Joaquin Valley that are still producing a commercial crop are over 75 years old. The life of the orchard at the time of planting is estimated to be 50 years.

3. <u>IRRIGATION:</u>

Pumped water (plus labor) is the irrigation cost. The cost is based on system pumping 24 acre-inches of water 350 feet in a 500-foot well over 500 acres. Water is pumped to the orchard after running through a filtration station into a permanent drip system in the tree rows. The cost of the irrigation system is for the installation of a new pump, well, filtration system, and permanent drip lines. The new irrigation system is installed after the orchard has been laid out and prior to planting. The life of the irrigation system is estimated at 30 years.

Price per acre foot of water will vary by grower in this region depending on power source, cost, various well characteristics, and other irrigation factors. In this study, water is estimated to cost $76.92 per acre foot. No assumption is made about effective rainfall. The amount of water applied to the orchard being established varies each year and is shown in **Table A.**

Table A. Applied Irrigation Water

Year	AcIn/Year
1	4
2	9
3	16
4	18
5+	24

1994 San Joaquin Valley Figs Cost and Return Study (Calimyrna Variety) UC Cooperative Extension 3

4. ESTABLISHMENT PRACTICES

This orchard is established on ground that has not been previously planted in trees or vines. The land is assumed to be slightly rolling and not on a Class I soil. The orchard site is not leveled, thus requiring a drip or sprinkler irrigation system.

Land Preparation: Land preparation begins with a deep ripping, going down 5 to 6 feet in order to break up underlying hardpans which would affect root and water penetration. The ripping is performed by contract operators. Following the ripping, the ground is disced then floated by the orchard owner. This breaks up large clods of soil and smoothes the ground in advance of planting the trees. All of the land preparation operations are done in the year prior to planting, but in this study, costs are shown in the first year.

Planting: Planting starts by marking the tree location with a stake. Then holes are dug and trees planted. The young trees are pruned back soon after planting. Regular pruning and sucker removal begins in the second year and hours and costs required to perform these tasks increase annually. Pruning is performed in the fall months. Removing the suckers is usually performed while weeding crews hand hoe the orchard. In the second year, 10 % of the trees or16 trees per acre will have to be replanted.

Orchard Floor Management: Weed control for the orchard begins in the fall with a residual herbicide sprayed along the tree rows. The same chemicals are used for this control during the life of the orchard, but only half of the full rate is used in the first two years; it is increased to the full rate in the third. In spring a contact herbicide is used to control vegetation in the middle of the tree rows with two applications. In the first two seasons, a full rate of the spot spray is used only on 25 percent of the acreage. Beginning in the third year, full rates are again used, but this time on a;; of the acreage. Discing is also used to control vegetation, and is performed four times during the first two years and once per season beginning in year three. Not only is discing used to manage orchard floor vegetation, but it also tills the soil in preparation for being packed, leveled, and smoothed. This operation produces a smooth, hard surface free of debris for efficient mechanical harvesting.

Pest Management: During typical years pest control in fig orchards is limited to controlling rodents, but in exceptionally cool weather a rapid build up of insect pests can occur which may require treatment. Baits are applied through the orchard at bait stations. Arthropod pests are typically not a problem in fig orchards, but serious infestations can occur and may require pest control. No insecticide or disease sprays are assumed to be used for the orchard in this study.

Fertilization: Nitrogen is the major nutrient required for proper tree growth and optimum fruit yields. Nitrogen fertilizer is spread in a granular form at increasing rates during orchard establishment and is shown in **Table B.**

Table B. Applied Nitrogen

Year	Pounds of N/Acre
1	10
2	20
3	30
4	40
5	50

1994 San Joaquin Valley Figs Cost and Return Study (Calimyrna Variety) UC Cooperative Extension 4

Pollination: Caprification or pollination of the figs occurs once a year in late May or early June and is supplemented by additional wasps contracted from an outside pollinator service. For further information see Pollination in the Production Cultural Practices section.

Establishment Cost: The cost to establish the orchard is used to determine the non-cash overhead expenses, depreciation and interest on investment, for the production years. The establishment cost is the sum of the costs for land preparation, planting, trees, cash overhead and production expenses for growing the trees through the first year that fruit is harvested. The *Total Accumulated Net Cash Cost* in the third year shown on **Table 1**, represents the establishment cost. For this study, this cost is $1,996 per acre or $828,340 for the 500 acres of mature orchard is estimated: this cost is shown in **Table 5**. This cost is spread over the remaining 47 years of the 50 years that the orchard is assumed to be in production.

5. PRODUCTION CULTURAL PRACTICES:

Pruning: Pruning is done by hand in the winter months. Prunings are pushed out of the orchard by a tractor using a brush rake and burned. Suckers are removed by hand crews as they hoe weeds during April.

Fertilization: Nitrogen fertilizer is applied in summer/fall following harvest. Proper levels of nitrogen to be applied to the orchard are determined by leaf analysis. Sampling is usually done in July, before the application of fertilizer. In this study, nitrogen is applied at a rate of 100 pounds per acre in the form of ammonium nitrate (34-0-0).

Orchard Floor Management: Weeds in the mature orchard are controlled with chemical and cultural practices as used in the later years of orchard establishment. A combination of residual herbicides is sprayed in a strip along the tree rows to control weeds there throughout the season. Tree row middles are disced once in the spring, to manage resident vegetation on the orchard floor and to prepare the ground to be packed, leveled, and smoothed prior to the first harvest. Vegetation in row middles that are not controlled by cultivation receives two sprays of a contact herbicide during spring and summer.

Pollination: Caprification refers to the pollination of Smyna type figs, such as the Calimyrna variety, by the wasp specie (Blastophaga psenes L.) This wasp performs the function that bees and other pollinators normally provide, by crawling across the male flower (also known as a caprifig), covering itself with pollen, a then entering the eye of the female fig (called the Calimyrna fig) and dusting the flowers with pollen. Typically the fig wasp is put out in the orchard during June.Fig wasps are usually supplied to the orchard during these periods in order to ensure proper pollination and good fruit set. In this study, services for caprification are provided by another fig grower or company that supplies the wasps at an annual cost of $60 per acre.

Pest Management: Arthropod and disease pests are commonly not serious enough in fig orchards to warrant treatment. The only pests that require control in this study are rodents. Commercially available baits are used in bait stations within the orchard in order to manage them during the growing season.

The pesticides and rates mentioned in this cost study are a few of those that are listed in the UC IPM Fig Pest Management Guidelines. Written recommendations are required for most pesticides and are made by licensed pest advisors. For information and pesticide use permits, contact the local county Agricultural Commission's office. For additional information contact the farm advisor of interest.

6. HARVEST:

Harvesting may start in the third or fourth year after the orchard is planted. As the yields increase, the cost to harvest also increases, until yield maturity is reached in the tenth year. The number of harvests per year also changes as the orchard matures. In the third year, three harvests are performed. The fourth year requires four, the fifth year, figs are harvested five times, and from the sixth year on six harvests are completed annually. In this cost study, the crop is harvested and sorted by the grower, although some growers custom hire the harvest operation.

Fig harvesting begins as the fruit naturally falls to the ground. In the late season crop some figs may cling to the trees, which require growers to use blowers to force those remaining fruit to fall. The sweeper windrows the figs into the middle of the orchard row so that the harvester can pick up the fruit and dump them into field bins. A hand crew may rake the figs that are lying next to the tree out to where a mechanical orchard sweeper can reach them. The figs are hauled from the field to a dry yard. A grower with 500 acres of figs in production is assumed to own his dry yard, and would sort his figs. After sorting, the figs are sold to processors.

For growers that do not own harvesting and packing equipment, the needed equipment for harvesting and packing operations should be removed from the equipment and investment inventories on **Table 5**, and custom harvest and packing charges should be placed in Harvest costs in **Table 1** and **2**, to replace grower performed harvest and packing costs.

7. ASSESSMENTS:

Under a state marketing order, mandatory assessment fees are collected by the California Fig Advisory Board (CFAB). These assessments are charged both to the grower and the processor to pay for fig marketing and advertising. Half of the fee of $48 per ton of merchantable fruit (merchantable fruit is destined for dried or paste markets) is paid by the grower and is shown in this study, while the remaining $24 is paid by the processor. Additionally, a voluntary assessment is also paid by fig growers for research and administration and is managed by the California Fig Institute (CFI). Though the assessment is voluntary it is currently supported by all of the growers. CFI charges growers $5 per ton of merchantable fruit. Both of these assessments are shown as a harvest cost.

8. YIELDS AND RETURNS

Yields: As noted above, figs most often begin bearing an economic crop in the third year after planting. Typical annual yields for the Calimyrna variety is measured in pounds merchantable figs and tons for cull fruit. Normal cull percentages for Calimyrna figs has decreased over the past ten years from a historical average of 27 to 15 percent, which resulted in increasing the amount of figs sold for higher value paste or dried fruit. This study uses a 16 percent cull rate. The yields shown in **Table C** are from the third year of orchard establishment to maturity.

Table C — Annual Yield Per Acre - Calimyrna

		Figs – Pounds/Acre		
Year	Tons/Acre	Total	Merchantable	Cull
3	0.10	200	168	32
4	0.20	400	336	64
5	0.40	800	672	128
6	0.55	1,100	924	176
7	0.65	1,300	1,092	208
8	0.80	1,600	1,344	256
9	0.85	1,700	1,445	255
10+	0.90	1,800	1,520	280

1994 San Joaquin Valley Figs Cost and Return Study (Calimyrna Variety) UC Cooperative Extension 6

Returns Calimyrna figs command higher prices than either the Black Mission or Conadria varieties. Return prices for Calimyrnas over the past ten years have ranged from $0.35 to over $1.00 per pound of merchantable fruit. For figs that are sold for dried fruit or paste a price of $0.80 per pound is used. Culled fruit is sold for cattle feed with the grower receiving $0.03 per pound in this study. **Table** 7 indicates returns to risk and management at various levels of fig prices and yields. It calculates returns above three levels of cost: operating, cash and total.

9. RISK:

Risk is caused by various sources of uncertainty which include production, price, and financial. Examples of these are insect damage, a decrease in price, and increase in interest rates. The risks associated with fig production should not be underestimated. While this study makes every effort to model a production system based on typical, real world practices, it cannot fully represent financial, agronomic and market risks which affect the profitability and economic viability of fig production. Due to the risk involved, access to a market is crucial. A market channel should be determined before any fig orchards are planted and brought into production.

10. LABOR:

Basic hourly wages for workers are $6.00 and $4.51 per hour for machine operators and field workers (irrigator), respectively. Adding 34 percent for Workers Compensation, Social Security, Medicare, insurance and other benefits gives the labor rates shown of $8.04 per hour for machine labor and $6.04 per hour for non-machine labor. The labor hours for operations involving machinery are 20 percent higher than the machine hour; to account for extra labor involved in equipment set-up, moving, maintenance, and repair. Wages for mangers are not included as a cash cost. Any returns above total costs are considered returns to investment.

11. CASH OVERHEAD:

Cash overhead consists of various cash expenses paid out during the year assigned to the whole farm and not to a particular operation. These costs include property taxes, interest on operating capital, office expense, liability and property insurance, sanitation services, and investment repairs.

Property Tax: Counties charge a base property tax rate of 1 percent on the assessed value of the property. In some counties special assessment districts exist and charge additional taxes on property including equipment, buildings, and improvements. County taxes are calculated as 1 percent of the average value of the property for this study. Average value equals new cost plus salvage value divided by two on a per acre basis.

Interest On Operating Capital: Interest on operating capital is based on cash operating costs and is calculated monthly until harvest at a nominal rate of 7.89 percent per year. A nominal interest rate is the going market cost of borrowed funds.

Office Expense: Office and business expenses are estimated at $100 per acre. These expenses include office supplies, telephones, bookkeeping, accounting, legal fees, and road maintenance.

Insurance: Insurance for farm investments vary depending on the assets covered and the amount of coverage. Property insurance provides coverage for property loss and is charged at 0.713 percent of the average value of the assets over their useful life. Liability insurance covers accidents on the farm, and costs $330 for the entire farm or $0.66 per acre.

Sanitation: Sanitation services provide portable toilets for the orchard and cost the farm $970 annually. Cash overhead costs are found in **Tables 1, 2, 3, 4** and **5.**

12. NON-CASH OVERHEAD:

Non-cash overhead is comprised of depreciation and interest charged on equipment and other investments. Most of the equipment inventory in typical fig orchards in the San Joaquin Valley is purchased both new and used. This study shows current purchase price for new equipment adjusted to 60 percent of new value to indicate a mix of new and used equipment. Annual equipment and investment costs are shown in **Tables 1, 2,** and **5**. They represent depreciation and opportunity cost for each investment on an annual per acre basis.

Depreciation: Depreciation is a reduction in market value of investments due to wear, obsolescence, and age, and is on a straight line basis. Annual depreciation is calculated as purchase price minus salvage value divided by years the investment is held. The purchase price and years of life are shown in **Table 5.**

Opportunity Costs: Interest is charged on investments to account for income foregone (opportunity cost) that could be received from an alternative investment. The investments are assumed to be owned outright. Therefore, interest on investments is a non-cash cost. Investments include land, orchard, buildings, and equipment. Interest is calculated as the average value of the investment during its useful life, multiplied by 3.72 percent per year. Average value for equipment and buildings equals new cost plus salvage value divided by two on a per acre basis. The average value for land is equal to the purchase price because land does not depreciate. Real interest rates are used on long term assets to show current costs.

13. EQUIPMENT CASH COSTS:

Equipment costs are composed of three parts; non-cash overhead, cash overhead, and operating costs. Both of the overhead factors have been discussed in previous sections. The operating costs consist of fuel, lubrication, and repairs.

In allocating the equipment costs on a per acre basis, the following hourly charges are calculated first and shown in **Table 6.** Repair costs are based on purchase price, annual hours of use, total hours of life, and repair coefficients formulated by the American Society of Agricultural Engineers (ASAE). Fuel and lubrication costs are also determined by ASAE equations based on maximum PTO hp, and type of fuel used. The fuel and repair cost per acre for each operation in **Table 2** is determined by multiplying the total hourly operating cost in **Table 6** for each piece of equipment used for the cultural practice by the number of hours per acre for that operation. Tractor time is 10 percent higher than implement time for a given operation to account for setup time. Prices for on-farm delivery of diesel and gasoline are $0.85 and $1.17 per gallon, respectively.

14. ACKNOWLEDGMENT:

Appreciation is expressed to the California Fig Advisory Board, California Fig Institute, and several fig growers in the San Joaquin Valley who participated in this study. Their generously provided information and expertise helped make the production of this study possible.

REFERENCES

1. American Society of Agricultural Engineers. 1992. American Society of Agricultural Engineers Standards Yearbook. St. Joseph, MI.

2. Boelje, Michael D., and Vernon R. Eidman. 1984. Farm Management. John Wiley and Sons. New York, NY.

3. Obenauf, Gary, Marvin Gerdts, George Leavitt, and Julian Crane. 1978. Commercial Dried Fig Production in California. Leaflet 21051. UC DANR. Oakland, CA.

4. Statewide IPM Project. 1990. UC Pest management guidelines, alfalfa. In, UC IPM Pest Management Guidelines. Pub. 3339. UC DANR. Oakland, CA.

1994 San Joaquin Valley Fig Cost and Return Study (Calimyra Variety) UC Cooperative Extension 8

table 1.

U.C. COOPERATIVE EXTENSION
SAMPLE COSTS PER ACRE TO ESTABLISH A FIG ORCHARD
SAN JOAQUIN VALLEY - 1994
CALIMYRNA VARIETY

Labor Rate: $8.04/hr. machine labor — Trees Per Acre: 155
$6.04/hr. non-machine labor — Long Term Interest Rate: 3.72%

	Cost Per Acre				
Year	1st	2nd	3rd	4th	5th
Yield: Field Run - Pounds Per Acre			200	400	800
Planting Costs:					
Deep Rip - Custom	$300				
Disc	$4				
Float	$4				
Trees: 155 Per Acre @ $2.50	$388	$40			
Mark, Stake, Dig Holes & Plant - Contract	$78				
Replants: 10% in 2nd Year		$8			
TOTAL PLANTING COSTS	$773	$48			
Cultural Costs:					
Prune & Train	$46	$38	$57	$76	$85
Remove Brush	$7	7	7	7	7
Apply Fertilizer - Nitrogen	$6	10	14	18	21
Irrigate	$35	71	141	159	212
Caprification			$30	35	60
Pest Control - Rodents	$6	6	6	6	6
Weed Control - Disc Row Middles	$13	13	3	50	50
Smooth & Level Orchard Floor			$6	6	6
Weed Control - Hand Hoe and Remove Suckers	$12	12	12	12	12
Weed Control - Spray Middles 2X	$9	9	29	29	29
Weed Control - Strip Spray Residual	$51	51	64	64	64
Pickup Truck Use	$7	7	7	7	7
TOTAL CULTURAL COSTS	$194	$224	$378	$470	$560
Harvest Costs:					
Hand Knock Fruit			$3	$4	$5
Windrow Fruit			20	27	34
Pick Up Fruit			42	59	94
Haul To Shed			2	6	8
Sort Figs			12	24	48
Marketing Order Assessment Fee			2	5	10
Research & Administration Assessment Fee			1	1	2
TOTAL HARVEST COSTS			$82	$126	$201

1994 San Joaquin Valley Fig Cost and Return Study(Calimyrna Variety) — *UC Cooperative Extension*

U.C. COOPERATIVE EXTENSION
CALIMYRNA VARIETY
Table 1. continued

	Cost Per Acre				
Year	1st	2nd	3rd	4th	5th
Yield: Field Run - Pounds Per Acre			200	400	800
Interest On Operating Capital@ 7.89%	$25	$2	$4	$4	$5
Cash Overhead Costs:					
Office Expense	$101	$101	$101	$101	$101
Sanitation Fees	$2	2	2	2	2
Leaf Analysis	$5	5	5	5	5
Liability Insurance	$1	1	1	1	1
Property Taxes	$17	17	18	19	19
Property Insurance	$12	12	13	13	14
Investment Repairs	$3	3	3	3	3
TOTAL CASH OVERHEAD COSTS	$142	$142	$144	$144	$145
TOTAL CASH COSTS	$1,134	$416	$607	$744	$911
INCOME FROM PRODUCTION			$160	$320	$640
NET CASH COSTS FOR THE YEAR	$1,134	$416	$447	$424	$271
ACCUMULATED NET CASH COSTS	$1,134	$1,549	$1,996	$2,420	$2,690
Depreciation:					
Shop Building	$3	$3	$3	$3	$3
Packing Shed	$23	23	23	23	23
Drip Irrigation System	$9	9	9	9	9
Shop Tools	$1	1	1	1	1
Fuel Tanks & Pumps	$1	1	1	1	1
Equipment	$13	11	32	37	47
TOTAL DEPRECIATION	$49	$47	$68	$73	$83
Interest On Investment @ 4.00%					
Shop Building	$2	$2	$2	$2	$2
Packing Shed	$10	10	10	10	10
Shop Tools	$4	4	4	4	4
Drip Irrigation System	$1	1	1	1	1
Fuel Tanks & Pumps	$1	1	1	1	1
Land @ $1500/Acre	$45	45	45	45	45
Equipment	$3	3	8	9	12
TOTAL INTEREST ON INVESTMENT	$65	$64	$70	$71	$74
TOTAL COST FOR THE YEAR	$1,248	$528	$744	$888	$1,067
INCOME FROM PRODUCTION			$160	$320	$640
TOTAL NET COST FOR THE YEAR	$1,248	$528	$584	$568	$427
TOTAL ACCUMULATED NET COST	$1,248	$1,775	$2,359	$2,928	$3,355

1994 San Joaquin Valley Fig Cost and Return Study(Calimyrna Variety) *UC Cooperative Extension*

Table 2.

U.C. COOPERATIVE EXTENSION
COSTS PER ACRE TO PRODUCE FIGS
SAN JOAQUIN VALLEY - 1994
CALIMYRNA VARIETY

Labor Rate: $8.04/hr. machine labor; $6.04/hr. non-machine labor
Interest Rate: 7.89 %
Yield per Acre: 1,800 Lb

Operation	Operation Time (Hrs/A)	Cash and Labor Costs per Acre: Labor Cost	Fuel/Lube & Repairs	Material Cost	Custom/ Rent	Total Cost	Your Cost
Cultural:							
Irrigate	9.60	57.98	0.00	141.02	0.00	199.00	
Prune And Train	14.00	84.56	0.00	0.00	0.00	84.56	
Clear Brush	0.14	2.76	1.67	0.00	0.00	4.43	
Fertilize - Nitrogen	0.16	1.54	0.88	18.45	0.00	20.87	
Weed Control - Disc Middles	0.20	1.93	1.41	0.00	0.00	3.34	
Smooth & Level Orchard Floor	0.33	3.22	2.33	0.00	0.00	5.54	
Hand Hoe And Remove Suckers	2.00	12.08	0.00	0.00	0.00	12.08	
Weed Control - Spray Middles 2X	0.15	1.48	0.38	27.32	0.00	29.18	
Pest Control - Rodents	0.50	0.48	0.12	5.80	0.00	6.41	
Caprification	0.00	0.00	0.00	0.00	60.00	60.00	
Weed Control - Strip Spray	0.25	2.37	1.66	60.12	0.00	64.16	
Pickup Truck Use	0.57	5.50	3.69	0.00	0.00	9.19	
TOTAL CULTURAL COSTS	27.46	173.91	12.13	252.72	60.00	498.76	
Harvest:							
Hand Knock Trees	1.00	6.04	0.00	0.00	0.00	6.04	
Windrow Fruit	0.38	14.48	16.72	0.00	0.00	31.20	
Pick Up Fruit	1.40	26.05	55.01	0.00	24.00	105.06	
Haul To Shed	0.00	0.00	0.00	0.00	18.00	18.00	
Sort Figs	0.00	0.00	0.00	162.00	0.00	162.00	
TOTAL HARVEST COSTS	2.78	46.57	71.73	162.00	42.00	322.30	
Assessments:							
Marketing Order	0.00	0.00	0.00	21.60	0.00	21.60	
Research & Administration	0.00	0.00	0.00	4.50	0.00	4.50	
TOTAL ASSESSMENT COSTS	0.00	0.00	0.00	26.10	0.00	26.10	

1994 San Joaquin Valley Fig Cost and Return Study(Calimyrna Variety) *UC Cooperative Extension*

U.C. COOPERATIVE
EXTENSION
CALIMYRNA VARIETY
Table 2. continued

TOTAL OPERATING COSTS/ACRE	220.48	83.87	440.82	102.00	867.83
TOTAL OPERATING COSTS/LB					0.57
CASH OVERHEAD:					
Office Expense					101.01
Leaf Analysis					4.55
Sanitation Fees					1.96
Liability Insurance					0.67
Property Taxes					30.30
Property Insurance					21.60
Investment Repairs					3.11
TOTAL CASH OVERHEAD COSTS					163.20
TOTAL CASH COSTS/ACRE					1,031.03
TOTAL CASH COSTS/LB					0.68

NON-CASH OVERHEAD:

Investment	Per producing Acre	Annual Cost: Depreciation	Annual Cost: Interest@3.72%	
Land	1,212.12		45.09	45.09
Packing Shed	505.05	22.73	10.33	33.06
Drip Irrigation System	202.83	9.13	4.15	13.28
Buildings	76.99	2.77	1.58	4.35
Shop Tools	22.89	1.37	0.47	1.84
Fuel Tanks & Pumps	12.84	0.58	0.26	0.84
Orchard Establishment	1,996.00	35.93	40.84	76.77
Equipment	488.55	42.34	10.00	52.33
TOTAL NON-CASH OVERHEAD COSTS	4,517.26	114.84	112.71	227.56
TOTAL COSTS/ACRE				1,258.58
TOTAL COSTS/LB				0.83

1994 San Joaquin Valley Fig Cost and Return Study(Calimyrna Variety) *UC Cooperative Extension*

Table 3.

U.C. COOPERATIVE EXTENSION
COSTS AND RETURNS PER ACRE TO PRODUCE FIGS
SAN JOAQUIN VALLEY - 1994
CALIMYRNA VARIETY

	Quantity/Ac	Unit	Price or Cost/Unit	Value or Cost/Acre	Your Cost
GROSS RETURNS					
Paste Figs	1,520.00	Lb	0.80	1,216.00	
Cull Figs	280.00	Lb	0.03	8.40	
TOTAL GROSS RETURNS FOR FIGS				1,224.40	
OPERATING COSTS					
Irrigation:					
Water - Pumped	22.00	AcIn	6.41	141.02	
Fertilizer:					
Ammonium Nitrate	50.00	Lb of N	0.37	18.45	
Herbicide:					
Roundup	2.00	Qt	13.66	27.32	
Surflan 4 AS	1.25	Qt	22.76	28.45	
Goal 1.6E	1.25	Qt	25.34	31.67	
Rodenticide:					
Rodent Bait	2.00	Lb	2.90	5.80	
Contract:					
Caprification	1.00	Acre	60.00	60.00	
Haul Figs	1,800.00	Lb	0.01	18.00	
Rent:					
Bin Rental	24.00	Bin	1.00	24.00	
Harvest Labor:					
Sort Figs	1,800.00	Lb	0.09	162.00	
Assessments:					
Marketing	0.90	Ton	24.00	21.60	
Research & Administration	0.90	Ton	5.00	4.50	
Labor (machine)	6.99	Hrs	8.04	56.19	
Labor (non-machine)	27.20	Hrs	6.04	164.29	
Fuel - Gas	6.27	Gal	1.17	7.33	
Fuel - Diesel	25.51	Gal	0.85	21.68	
Lube				4.35	
Machinery repair				50.49	
Interest on Operating Capital @ 7.89%				20.67	
TOTAL OPERATING COSTS/ACRE				867.83	
TOTAL OPERATING COSTS/LB				0.57	

1994 San Joaquin Valley Fig Cost and Return Study(Calimyrna Variety) *UC Cooperative Extension*

U.C. COOPERATIVE EXTENSION
CALIMYRNA VARIETY
Table 3. continued

NET RETURNS ABOVE OPERATING COSTS	356.57
CASH OVERHEAD COSTS:	
Office Expense	101.01
Leaf Analysis	4.55
Sanitation Fees	1.96
Liability Insurance	0.67
Property Taxes	30.30
Property Insurance	21.60
Investment Repairs	3.11
TOTAL CASH OVERHEAD COSTS/ACRE	163.20
TOTAL CASH COSTS/ACRE	1,031.03
TOTAL CASH COSTS/LB	0.68

Table 4.

U.C. COOPERATIVE EXTENSION
MONTHLY CASH COSTS PER ACRE TO PRODUCE FIGS
SAN JOAQUIN VALLEY - 1994
CALIMYRNA VARIETY

Beginning JAN 94 Ending DEC 94	JAN 94	FEB 94	MAR 94	APR 94	MAY 94	JUN 94	JUL 94	AUG 94	SEP 94	OCT 94	NOV 94	DEC 94	TOTAL
Cultural:													
Irrigate	35.30	35.30	35.30		35.30	22.48	35.30						199.00
Prune And Train	42.28	42.28											84.56
Clear Brush		4.43											4.43
Fertilize - Nitrogen			20.87										20.87
Weed Control - Disc Middle			3.34										3.34
Smooth & Level Orchard Floor			5.54										5.54
Hand Hoe And Remove Suckers				6.04	6.04								12.08
Weed Control - Spray Middles				14.59		14.59							29.18
Pest Control - Rodents					6.41								6.41
Caprification					60.00								60.00
Weed Control - Strip Spray										64.16			64.16
Pickup Truck Use										0.77			9.19
TOTAL CULTURAL COSTS	78.35	82.78	65.82	21.40	108.52	37.84	36.07	0.77	0.77	64.92	0.77	0.77	498.76
Harvest:													
Hand Knock Trees								1.99	3.02	1.03			6.04
Windrow Fruit								10.40	10.40	10.40			31.20
Pick Up Fruit								35.02	35.02	35.02			105.06
Haul To Shed								5.94	9.00	3.06			18.00
Sort Figs										27.54			162.00
TOTAL HARVEST COSTS								106.81	138.44	77.05			322.30
Assessments:													
Marketing Order								7.20	10.80	3.60			21.60
Research & Administration										0.75			4.50
TOTAL ASSESSMENT COSTS								8.70	13.05	4.35			26.10
Interest on Operating Capital	0.52	1.06	1.49	1.63	2.35	2.60	2.83	3.60	4.60				20.67
TOTAL OPERATING COSTS/ACRE	78.86	83.84	67.32	23.03	110.86	40.44	38.90	119.88	156.85	146.32	0.77	0.77	867.83
TOTAL OPERATING COSTS/LB	0.05	0.06	0.04	0.02	0.07	0.03	0.03	0.08	0.10	0.10	0.00	0.00	0.57
OVERHEAD:													
Office Expense	8.42	8.42	8.42	8.42	8.42	8.42	8.42	8.42	8.42	8.42	8.42	8.42	101.01
Leaf Analysis			4.55										4.55
Sanitation Fees	0.20	0.20	0.20	0.20	0.20	0.20	0.20	0.20	0.20	0.20			1.96
Liability Insurance	0.67												0.67
Property Taxes		15.15					15.15						30.30
Property Insurance	21.60												21.60
Investment Repairs										0.26			
TOTAL CASH OVERHEAD COSTS	31.14	24.02	13.42	8.87	8.87	8.87	24.02	8.87	8.87	8.87	8.68	8.68	163.20
TOTAL CASH COSTS/ACRE	110.01	107.86	80.73	31.90	119.73	49.31	62.92	128.75	165.73	155.19	9.44	9.44	1,031.03
TOTAL CASH COSTS/LB	0.07	0.07	0.05	0.02	0.08	0.03	0.04	0.08	0.11	0.10	0.01	0.01	0.68

1994 San Joaquin Valley Fig Cost and Return Study(Calimyrna Variety) *UC Cooperative Extension*

Table 5. U.C. COOPERATIVE EXTENSION
WHOLE FARM ANNUAL EQUIPMENT, INVESTMENT, AND BUSINESS OVERHEAD COSTS
SAN JOAQUIN VALLEY - 1994
CALIMYRNA VARIETY

ANNUAL EQUIPMENT COSTS

				Non-Cash Overhead		Cash Overhead		
Yr	Description	Price	Yrs Life	Depre- ciation	Interest	Insur- ance	Taxes	Total
94	62 HP 2WD Tractor	25,492	15	1,529.53	521.56	99.97	140.21	2,291.27
94	62 HP 2WD Tractor	25,492	15	1,529.53	521.56	99.97	140.21	2,291.27
94	ATV 4WD & Sprayer	7,430	10	668.70	152.02	29.14	40.86	890.72
94	Bin Trailer	979	15	58.73	20.03	3.84	5.38	87.98
94	Bin Trailer	979	15	58.73	20.03	3.84	5.38	87.98
94	Bin Trailer	979	15	58.73	20.03	3.84	5.38	87.98
94	Bin Trailer	979	15	58.73	20.03	3.84	5.38	87.98
94	Bin Trailer	979	15	58.73	20.03	3.84	5.38	87.98
94	Bin Trailer	979	15	58.73	20.03	3.84	5.38	87.98
94	Brush Rake & Loader	6,000	25	216.00	122.76	23.53	33.00	395.29
94	Brush Rake & Loader	6,000	25	216.00	122.76	23.53	33.00	395.29
94	Disc - Tandem 14'	7,274	10	654.70	148.82	28.52	40.01	872.05
94	Forklift - 4 Ton	11,261	10	1,013.50	230.40	44.16	61.94	1,350.00
94	Forklift - 4 Ton	11,261	10	1,013.50	230.40	44.16	61.94	1,350.00
94	Orchard Leveler	13,889	15	833.33	284.17	54.47	76.39	1,248.36
94	Harvester - SP [1]	61,133	10	5,502.00	1,250.78	239.73	336.23	7,328.74
94	Harvester - SP [1]	61,133	10	5,502.00	1,250.78	239.73	336.23	7,328.74
94	Harvester - SP [1]	61,133	10	5,502.00	1,250.78	239.73	336.23	7,328.74
94	Pick Up Truck 1/2 Ton	17,160	7	2,206.29	351.09	67.29	94.38	2,719.05
94	Spinner Spreader - 3 Pt	878	20	39.50	17.97	3.44	4.83	65.74
94	Sweeper - SP [1]	28,743	10	2,586.90	588.08	112.71	158.09	3,445.78
94	Sweeper - SP [1]	28,743	10	2,586.90	588.08	112.71	158.09	3,445.78
94	Sweeper - SP [1]	28,743	10	2,586.90	588.08	112.71	158.09	3,445.78
94	Weed Sprayer 100 Gal	3,550	10	319.50	72.63	13.92	19.52	425.57
TOTAL		411,189		34,859.16	8,412.90	1,612.46	2,261.53	47,146.05
60% of New Cost [2]		246,713		20,915.50	5,047.74	967.48	1,356.92	28,287.63

[1] SP = self propelled
[2] Used to reflect a mix of new and used equipment.

1994 San Joaquin Valley Fig Cost and Return Study(Calimyrna Variety) *UC Cooperative Extension*

U.C. COOPERATIVE EXTENSION
SAN JOAQUIN VALLEY - 1994
CALIMYRNA VARIETY
Table 5. continued

ANNUAL INVESTMENT COSTS

			Non-Cash Overhead			Cash Overhead		
Description	Price	Yrs Life	Depre-ciation	Interest	Insur-ance	Taxes	Repairs	Total
INVESTMENT								
Buildings	38,110	25	1,371.96	779.73	149.45	209.61	152.40	2,663.15
Orchard Establishment	828,340	50	14,910.10	16,947.80	3,248.34	4,555.87	0.00	39,662.11
Drip Irrigation System	100,400	20	4,518.00	2,054.18	393.72	552.20	150.00	7,668.10
Fuel Tanks & Pumps	6,355	20	285.95	130.03	24.92	34.96	125.00	600.86
Land	600,000	50		22,320.00	4,278.00	6,000.00	0.00	32,598.00
Packing Shed	250,000	20	11,250.00	5,115.00	980.37	1,375.00	1,000.00	19,720.37
Shop Tools	11,330	15	679.80	231.81	44.43	62.32	113.00	1,131.36
TOTAL INVESTMENT	1,834,535		33,015.81	47,578.55	9,119.23	12,789.96	1,540.40	104,043.95

ANNUAL BUSINESS OVERHEAD COSTS

Description	Units/ Farm	Unit	Price/ Unit	Total Cost
Leaf Analysis	500	Acre	4.50	2,250
Liability Insurance	500	Acre	0.66	330
Office Expense	500	Acre	100.00	50,000
Sanitation Fees	500	Acre	1.94	970

U.C. COOPERATIVE EXTENSION
SAN JOAQUIN VALLEY - 1994
CALIMYRNA VARIETY

Table 6. HOURLY EQUIPMENT COSTS

		COSTS PER HOUR							
	Actual	Non-Cash Overhead		Cash Overhead		Operating			
	Hours Used	Depreciation	Interest	Insurance	Taxes	Repairs	Fuel & Lube	Total Oper.	Total Costs
94 62 HP 2WD Tractor	799.2	1.15	0.39	0.08	0.11	1.53	2.98	4.51	6.23
94 62 HP 2WD Tractor	799.0	1.15	0.39	0.08	0.11	1.53	2.98	4.51	6.23
94 ATV 4WD & Sprayer	299.0	1.34	0.31	0.06	0.08	0.89	1.35	2.24	4.03
94 Bin Trailer	165.5	0.21	0.07	0.01	0.02	0.23	0.00	0.23	0.55
94 Bin Trailer	165.5	0.21	0.07	0.01	0.02	0.23	0.00	0.23	0.55
94 Bin Trailer	165.5	0.21	0.07	0.01	0.02	0.23	0.00	0.23	0.55
94 Bin Trailer	165.5	0.21	0.07	0.01	0.02	0.23	0.00	0.23	0.55
94 Bin Trailer	165.5	0.21	0.07	0.01	0.02	0.23	0.00	0.23	0.55
94 Bin Trailer	165.5	0.21	0.07	0.01	0.02	0.23	0.00	0.23	0.55
94 Brush Rake&Loader	99.3	1.30	0.74	0.14	0.20	0.87	0.00	0.87	3.26
94 Brush Rake & Loader	99.3	1.30	0.74	0.14	0.20	0.87	0.00	0.87	3.26
94 Disc - Tandem 14'	250.0	1.57	0.36	0.07	0.10	2.09	0.00	2.09	4.19
94 Forklift - 4 Ton	300.0	2.03	0.46	0.09	0.12	3.38	9.42	12.80	15.50
94 Forklift - 4 Ton	300.0	2.03	0.46	0.09	0.12	3.38	9.42	12.80	15.50
94 Orchard Leveler	165.3	3.02	1.03	0.20	0.28	2.02	0.00	2.02	6.55
94 Harvester - SP [1]	228.3	14.46	3.29	0.63	0.88	18.34	7.82	26.16	45.43
94 Harvester - SP [1]	228.3	14.46	3.29	0.63	0.88	18.34	7.82	26.16	45.43
94 Harvester - SP [1]	228.3	14.46	3.29	0.63	0.88	18.34	7.82	26.16	45.43
94 Pickup Truck 1/2 Ton	284.6	4.65	0.74	0.14	0.20	3.11	3.36	6.47	12.21
94 Spinner Spreader - 3 Pt	66.4	0.36	0.16	0.03	0.04	0.53	0.00	0.53	1.12
94 Sweeper - SP [1]	199.2	7.79	1.77	0.34	0.48	8.62	4.89	13.51	23.89
94 Sweeper - SP [1]	199.2	7.79	1.77	0.34	0.48	8.62	4.89	13.51	23.89
94 Sweeper - SP [1]	199.2	7.79	1.77	0.34	0.48	8.62	4.89	13.51	23.89
94 Weed Sprayer 100 Gal	119.1	1.61	0.37	0.07	0.10	1.78	0.00	1.78	3.93

[1] SP = self propelled

Table 7.

U.C. COOPERATIVE EXTENSION
RANGING ANALYSIS
SAN JOAQUIN VALLEY - 1994

COSTS PER ACRE AT VARYING YIELDS TO PRODUCE CALIMYRNA FIGS

	YIELD [1] (LB/ACRE)						
	500	1000	1500	2000	2500	3000	3500
OPERATING COSTS/ACRE:							
Cultural Cost	499	499	499	499	499	499	499
Harvest Cost	76	197	317	438	559	679	800
Assessment Cost	26	26	26	26	26	26	26
Interest on operating capital	19	20	21	21	22	23	24
TOTAL OPERATING COSTS/ACRE	620	742	863	984	1106	1227	1348
TOTAL OPERATING COSTS/LB	1.24	0.74	0.58	0.49	0.44	0.41	0.39
CASH OVERHEAD COSTS/ACRE	164	163	163	163	163	163	163
TOTAL CASH COSTS/ACRE	785	904	1026	1148	1269	1390	1512
TOTAL CASH COSTS/LB	1.57	0.90	0.68	0.57	0.51	0.46	0.43
NON-CASH OVERHEAD COSTS/ACRE	241	224	227	229	230	230	230
TOTAL COSTS/ACRE	1025	1128	1254	1376	1499	1621	1742
TOTAL COSTS/LB	2.05	1.13	0.84	0.69	0.60	0.54	0.50

[1] Yields are a combination of both paste and cull fig production.

NET RETURNS PER ACRE ABOVE OPERATING COSTS FOR CALIMYRNA FIGS

PRICE DOLLARS/POUND		YIELD [1] POUND/ACRE						
Merchantable		422	844	1,267	1,689	2,956	2,533	2,956
	Culls	78	156	233	311	389	467	544
0.50	0.03	-407	-315	-223	-130	383	54	146
0.60	0.03	-364	-231	-96	39	679	307	442
0.70	0.03	-322	-146	31	208	975	560	737
0.80	0.03	-280	-62	157	376	1,270	814	1,033
0.90	0.03	-238	23	284	545	1,566	1,067	1,328
1.00	0.03	-195	107	411	714	1,861	1,320	1,624
1.10	0.03	-153	192	537	883	2,157	1,574	1,919

1994 San Joaquin Valley Fig Cost and Return Study(Calimyrna Variety) *UC Cooperative Extension*

U.C. COOPERATIVE EXTENSION
Table 7. continued

NET RETURNS PER ACRE ABOVE CASH COSTS FOR CALIMYRNA FIGS

PRICE DOLLARS/POUND		YIELD [1] POUND/ACRE						
Merchantable		422	844	1,267	1,689	2,956	2,533	2,956
	Culls	78	156	233	311	389	467	544
0.50	0.03	-572	-477	-386	-294	220	-109	-18
0.60	0.03	-529	-393	-259	-125	516	144	278
0.70	0.03	-487	-308	-132	44	812	397	573
0.80	0.03	-445	-224	-6	212	1,107	651	869
0.90	0.03	-403	-139	121	381	1,403	904	1,164
1.00	0.03	-360	-55	248	550	1,698	1,157	1,460
1.10	0.03	-318	30	374	719	1,994	1,411	1,755

NET RETURNS PER ACRE ABOVE TOTAL COSTS FOR CALIMYRNA FIGS

PRICE DOLLARS/POUND		YIELD [1] POUND/ACRE						
Merchantable		422	844	1,267	1,689	2,956	2,533	2,956
	Culls	78	156	233	311	389	467	544
0.50	0.03	-812	-701	-614	-522	-10	-340	-248
0.60	0.03	-769	-617	-487	-353	286	-87	48
0.70	0.03	-727	-532	-360	-184	582	166	343
0.80	0.03	-685	-448	-234	-16	877	420	639
0.90	0.03	-643	-363	-107	153	1,173	673	934
1.00	0.03	-600	-279	20	322	1,468	926	1,230
1.10	0.03	-558	-194	146	491	1,764	1,180	1,525

[1] Yields are a combination of both paste and cull fig production.

1994 San Joaquin Valley Fig Cost and Return Study(Calimyrna Variety) *UC Cooperative Extension*

U.C COOPERATIVE EXTENSION

GENERAL ASSUMPTIONS FOR ESTABLISHING A FIG ORCHARD AND PRODUCING FIGS

Black Mission Variety - San Joaquin Valley - 1994

The following is a description of some general assumptions pertaining to sample costs of Black Mission variety fig establishment and production in the San Joaquin Valley. Practices described should not be considered recommendations by the University of California, but rather represent production procedures considered typical for this crop and area. Some of these costs and practices may not be applicable to your situation nor used during every production year Additional ones not indicated may be needed. Establishment and production practices for figs vary by grower and region and can be significant. The practices and inputs used in this cost study serve only as a sample or guide. These costs are represented on an annual, per acre basis. *The use of trade names in this report does not constitute an endorsement or recommendation by the University of California nor is any criticism implied by omission of other similar products*

1. LAND:

The farm consists of 500 acres of land. There are 80 acres currently being established in the actual fig orchard with another 415 acres on which figs are grown and 5 acres of roads and farmstead. No other crops are grown. Land is
valued at $1,200 per acre.

2. TREES:

The specific variety of fig trees planted in this study is Black Mission. The trees are planted at 15 x 20 foot spacing, with 155 trees per acre. Fig trees have a very long production life if well maintained. Some fig orchards in the San Joaquin Valley still producing a commercial crop are over 75 years old. The life of the orchard at the time of planting is estimated to be 50 years.

3. IRRIGATION:

Pumped water (plus labor) is the irrigation cost. The cost is based on system pumping 24 acre-inches of water 350 feet in a 500 foot well over 500 acres. Water is pumped to the orchard after running through a filtration station into a permanent drip system in the tree rows. The cost of the irrigation system is for the installation of a new pump, well, filtration system, and permanent drip lines. The new irrigation system is installed after the orchard has been laid out and prior to planting. The life of the irrigation system is estimated at 30 years.

Price per acre foot of water will vary by grower in this region depending on power source, cost, various well characteristics, and other irrigation factors. In this study, water is estimated to cost $76.92 per acre foot. No assumption is made about effective rainfall. The amount of water applied to the orchard being established varies each year and is shown in **Table A.**

Table A. Applied Irrigation Water

Year	AcIn/Year
1	4
2	9
3	16
4	18
5+	24

4. ESTABLISHMENT PRACTICES:

Orchard Development: This orchard is established on ground that has not been previously planted in trees or vines. The land is assumed to be slightly rolling and not on Class I soil. The orchard site is not leveled, thus requiring a drip or sprinkler irrigation system.

Land preparation begins with a deep ripping, going down five to six feet in order to break up underlying hardpans which would affect root and water penetration. The ripping is performed by contract operators. Following the ripping, the ground is first disced and then floated by the orchard owner. This helps to break up large clods of soil and smooth the ground in advance of planting the trees. All of the operations that prepare the orchard for planting are done in the first year.

Planting: Planting starts by marking the tree location with a stake. Holes are then dug and the trees are planted. The young trees are pruned back soon after planting. Regular pruning and sucker removal begin in the second year and hours required to perform these tasks as well may be factorized in as costs increase annually. Pruning is performed in the fall months. Removing the suckers is usually performed while weeding crews hand hoe the orchard. In the second year, 10 percent of the trees or 16 trees per acre will have to be replanted.

Orchard Floor Management: Weed control for the orchard begins in the fall with a residual herbicide sprayed along the tree rows. The same chemicals are used for this control during the life of the orchard, but only half of the full rate is used in the first two years and increases to the full rate in the third. In spring a contact herbicide is used to control vegetation in the middle of the tree rows with two applications. In the first two seasons, a full rate of the spot spray is used only on 25 percent of the acreage. Beginning in the third year, full rates are again used, but this time on all of the acreage. Discing is also used to control vegetation and is performed four times during the first two years and once per season from year three. Discing is not only used to manage orchard floor vegetation, but it also tills the soil in preparation for being packed, leveled, and smoothed. This operation produces a smooth, hard surface free of debris for efficient mechanical harvesting.

Pest Management: Pest control in fig orchards is limited to controlling rodents. Baits are applied through the orchard at bait stations. Arthropod pests are typically not a problem in fig orchards, but serious infestations can occur and may require pest control. No insecticide or disease sprays are assumed to be used for the orchard in this study.

Fertilization: Nitrogen is the major nutrient required for proper tree growth and optimum fruit yields. Nitrogen fertilizer is spread in a granular form of ammonium nitrate (34-0-0) at increasing rates during orchard establishment and is shown in **Table B.**

Table B. Applied Nitrogen

Year	Pounds Of N/ Acre
1	20
2	40
3	60
4	80
5+	100

Establishment Cost: The cost to establish the orchard is used to determine the non-cash overhead expenses, depreciation and interest on investment, for the production years. The establishment cost is the sum of the costs for land preparation, planting, trees, cash overhead and production expenses for growing the trees through the first year that fruit is harvested. The *Total Accumulated Net Cash Cost*

1994 San Joaquin Valley Figs Cost and Return Study (Black Mission Variety) UC Cooperative Extension 4

shown on **Table 1 (This and all subsequent Tables can be found on the UC Davis Cooperative Extension website)**, in the third year represents the establishment cost. For this study, this cost is $2,059 per acre or $854,485 for the 415 acres of mature orchard is estimated: this cost is shown in **Table 5**. The establishment cost is spread over the remaining 47 years of the 50 years that the orchard is assumed to be in production.

5. PRODUCTION CULTURAL PRACTICES:

Pruning: Pruning is done by hand in the winter months. Prunings are pushed out of the orchard by a tractor using a brush rake and burned. Suckers are removed by hand crews as they hoe weeds during April.

Fertilization: Nitrogen fertilizer is applied in summer/fall following harvest. Proper levels of nitrogen to be applied to the orchard are determined by leaf analysis. Sampling is usually done in July, prior to the application of fertilizer. Nitrogen is applied at a rate of 100 pounds of N per acre.

Orchard Floor Management: Weeds in the mature orchard are controlled with chemical and cultural practices as used in the later years of orchard establishment. A combination of residual herbicides is sprayed in a strip along the tree rows to control weeds there throughout the season. Tree row middles are disced once in the spring to manage resident vegetation on the orchard floor and to prepare the ground to be packed, leveled, and smoothed prior to the first harvest. Vegetation in row middles that are not controlled by cultivation receive two sprays of a contact herbicide during spring and summer.

Insect And Disease Management: Arthropods and disease pests are commonly not serious enough in a well managed fig orchard to warrant treatment. The only pests that require control in this study are rodents. Commercially available baits are used in bait stations within the orchard in order to manage them during the growing season.

The pesticides and rates mentioned in this cost study are a few of those that are listed in the UC IPM Fig Pest Management Guidelines. Written recommendations are required for most pesticides and are made by licensed pest control advisors. For information and pesticide use permits, contact the local county Agricultural Commissioner's office. For additional information contact the farm advisor in the county of interest.

6. HARVEST:

Harvesting starts in the third year after the orchard is planted. The number of times that the orchard is harvested changes in each year. In the third year the orchard is harvested three times; in the fourth year, four times; the fifth year, five times and from the sixth year on, figs are harvested six times per year. As the yields increase, the cost to harvest also increases until maturity is reached in the tenth year. In this cost study the crop is harvested and sorted by the grower.

Fig harvesting begins as the fruit naturally falls to the ground. In the late season crop some figs may cling to the trees, which require growers to use blowers to force those remaining fruit to fall. The sweeper windrows the figs into the middle of the orchard row so that the harvester can pick up the fruit and dump them into field bins. A hand crew may rake the figs that are lying next to the tree out to where a mechanical orchard sweeper can reach them. The figs are hauled from the field to a dry yard. A grower with 500 acres of figs in production is assumed to own their dry yard and would sort their figs. After sorting, the figs are sold to processors.

For growers that do not own harvesting and packing equipment, the needed equipment for harvesting and packing operations should be removed from the equipment and investment inventories on **Table 5**,

1994 San Joaquin Valley Figs Cost and Return Study (Black Mission Variety) UC Cooperative Extension 5

and custom harvest and packing charges should be placed in Harvest costs in **Tables 1** and 2. All of the grower performed harvest and packing costs would be subtracted from Harvest costs given in **Tables 1** and 2. (These tables are available in the complete study at UCCooperative Extension.

7. <u>ASSESSMENTS:</u>

Under a state marketing order, mandatory assessment fees are collected by the California Fig Advisory Board (CFAB). These assessments are charged both to the grower and the processor to pay for fig marketing and advertising. Half of the fee of $48 per ton of merchantable fruit (merchantable fruit is destined for dried, or paste markets) is paid by the grower and is shown in this study, while the remaining $24 is paid by the processor. Additionally, a voluntary assessment is also paid by fig growers for research and administration and is managed by the California Fig Institute (CFI). Though the assessment is voluntary it is currently supported by 100 % of the growers. CFI charges growers $5 per ton of merchantable fruit. Both of these assessments are shown as a harvest cost.

8. <u>YIELDS AND RETURNS:</u>

Yields: As noted above, figs most often begin bearing an economic crop in the third year after planting. Typical annual yields for the Black Mission variety is measured in pounds for paste figs and pounds and/or tons for cull fruit. Typical cull percentages for Black Mission figs have ranged between 3-6 percent. This study uses a 6 percent cull rate. The yields shown in **Table C** are from the third year of orchard establishment to maturity.

Table C — **Annual Yield Per Acre**

		Figs – Pounds/Acre		
Year	Tons/Acre	Total	Merchantable	Cull
3	0.20	400	372	28
4	0.80	1,600	1,488	112
5	1.20	2,400	2,232	168
6	1.52	3,040	2,827	213
7	1.80	3,600	3,348	252
8	2.00	4,000	3,720	280
9	2.24	4,480	4,166	314
10+	2.40	4,800	4,464	336

Returns: Black Mission figs are used in the dried or paste markets. For Black Mission figs sold for dried fruit or paste, a price of $0.50 per pound is used. Culled fruit is sold for cattle feed with the grower receiving $0.03 per pound in this study. **Table** 7 indicates returns to risk and management at various levels of fig categories, prices and yields. It calculates returns above three levels of cost: operating, cash and total.

9. <u>RISK:</u>

Risk is caused by various sources of uncertainty which include production, price, and financial. Examples of these are insect damage, a decrees in price, and increase in interest rates. The risks associated with fig production should not be underestimated. While this study makes every effort to model a production system based on typical, real world practices, it cannot fully represent financial, agronomic and market risks which affect the profitability and economic viability of fig production. Due to the risk involved, access to a market is crucial. A market channel should be determined before any fig orchards are planted and brought into production.

10. <u>LABOR:</u>

Basic hourly wages for workers are $6.00 and $4.51 per hour for machine operators and field workers (irrigation), respectively. Adding 34 percent for Workers Compensation, Social Security, Medicare, insurance and other benefits gives the labor rates shown of $8.04 per hour for machine labor and $6.04 per hour for non-machine labor. The labor hours for operations involving machinery are 20 percent higher

1994 San Joaquin Valley Figs Cost and Return Study (Black Mission Variety) UC Cooperative Extension 6

than the machine hours to account for extra labor involved in equipment set-up, moving, maintenance and repair. Wages for managers are not included as a cash cost. Any returns above total costs are considered returns to investment.

10. CASH OVERHEAD:

Cash overhead consists of various cash expenses paid out during the year that are assigned to the whole farm and not to a particular operation. These costs include property taxes, interest on operating capital, office expense, liability and property insurance, sanitation services, leaf analysis, and investment repairs.

Property Tax: Counties charge a base property tax rate of 1 on the assessed value of the property. In some counties special assessment districts exist and charge additional taxes on property including equipment, buildings, and improvements. County taxes are calculated as 1 percent of the average value of the property for this study. Average value equals new cost plus salvage value divided by two on a per acre basis.

Interest On Operating Capital: Interest on operating capital is based on cash operating costs and is calculated monthly until harvest at a nominal rate of 7.89 percent per year. A nominal interest rate is the going market cost of borrowed funds.

Office Expense: Office and business expenses are estimated at $100 per acre. These expenses include office supplies, telephone service, bookkeeping, accounting, legal fees, road maintenance, etc.

Insurance: Insurance for farm investments vary depending on the assets covered and the amount of coverage. Property insurance provides coverage for property loss and is charged at 0.713 percent of the average value of the assets over their useful life. Liability insurance covers accidents on the farm and costs $615 for the entire farm or $1.23 per acre.

Sanitation Services: Sanitation services provide portable toilets for the orchard and cost the farm $970 annually. The cost for this includes delivery and servicing of field toilets.

Leaf Analysis: Analysis for nutrients needed for proper tree growth and fruit development is performed on leaf petiole samples. A cost of $4.50 per acre covers this service. Many fertilization programs are based in part on leaf analysis. Cash overhead costs are found in **Tables 1, 2, 3, 4,** and **5**.

12. NON-CASH OVERHEAD:

Non-cash overhead is comprised of depreciation and interest charged on equipment and other investments. Most of the equipment inventory in typical fig orchards in the San Joaquin Valley is purchased both new and used. This study shows current purchase price for new equipment adjusted to 60 percent of new value to indicate a mix of new and used equipment. Annual equipment and investment costs are shown in **Tables 1, 2,** and **5**. They represent depreciation and opportunity cost for each investment on an annual per acre basis.

Depreciation: Depreciation is a reduction in market value of investments due to wear, obsolescence, and age, and is on a straight line basis. Annual depreciation is calculated as purchase price minus salvage value divided by years the investment is held. The purchase price and years of life are shown in **Table 5**.

Opportunity Costs: Interest is charged on investments to account for income foregone (opportunity cost) that could be received from an alternative investment. The investments are assumed to be owned outright. Therefore, interest on investments is a non-cash cost. Investments include land, orchard,

1994 San Joaquin Valley Figs Cost and Return Study (Black Mission Variety) UC Cooperative Extension 7

buildings, and equipment. Interest is calculated as the average value of the investment during its useful life, multiplied by 3.72 percent per year. Average value for equipment and buildings equals new cost plus salvage value divided by two on a per acre basis. The average value for land is equal to the purchase price because land does not depreciate. Real interest rates are used on long term assets to show current costs.

13. EQUIPMENT CASH COSTS:

Equipment costs are composed of three parts; non-cash overhead, cash overhead, and operating costs. The operating costs consist of fuel, lubrication, and repairs.

In allocating the equipment costs on a per acre basis, the following hourly charges are calculated first and shown in **Table 6.** Repair costs are based on purchase price, annual hours of use, total hours of life, and repair coefficients formulated by the American Society of Agricultural Engineers (ASAE). Fuel and lubrication costs are also determined by ASAE equations based on maximum PTO hp, and type of fuel used. The fuel and repair cost per acre for each operation in **Table 2** is determined by multiplying the total hourly operating cost in **Table 6** for each piece of equipment used for the cultural practice by the number of hours per acre for that operation. Tractor time is 10 percent higher than implement time for a given operation to account for setup time. Prices for on-farm delivery of diesel and gasoline are $0.85 and $1.17 per gallon, respectively.

14. ACKNOWLEDGMENT:

Appreciation is expressed to the California Fig Advisory Board, California Fig Institute, and the fig growers in the San Joaquin Valley who participated in this study. Their generously provided information and expertise helped make the production of this study possible.

REFERENCES

1. American Society of Agricultural Engineers. 1992. American Society of Agricultural Engineers Standards Yearbook. St. Joseph, MI.

2. Boelje, Michael D., and Vernon R. Eidman. 1984. Farm Management. John Wiley and Sons. New York, NY.

3. Obenauf, Gary, Marvin Gerdts, George Leavitt, and Julian Crane. 1978. Commercial Dried Fig Production in California. Leaflet 21051. UC DANR. Oakland, CA.

4. Statewide IPM Project. 1990. UC Pest management guidelines, alfalfa. In, UC IPM Pest Management Guidelines. Pub. 3339. UC DANR. Oakland, CA.

1994 San Joaquin Valley Figs Cost and Return Study (Black Mission Variety) UC Cooperative Extension 8

U.C. COOPERATIVE EXTENSION

GENERAL ASSUMPTIONS
FOR ESTABLISHING A FIG ORCHARD AND PRODUCING FIGS
Conadria Variety - San Joaquin Valley - 1994

The following contains some general assumptions pertaining to sample costs of conadria variety fig establishment and production in the San Joaquin Valley. Practices described should not be considered recommendations by the University of California, but rather represent production procedures considered typical for this crop and area. Some of these costs and practices may not be applicable to your situation nor used during every production year. Additional ones not indicated may be needed. Establishment and cultural practices for the production of figs vary by grower and region. The practices and inputs used in this cost study serve only as a sample or guide. Variations can be significant. These costs are represented on an annual, per acre basis. *The use of trade names in this report does not constitute an endorsement or recommendation by the University of California nor is any criticism implied by omission of other similar products.*

1. LAND:

The farm consists of 500 acres of land. There are 80 acres currently being established in the actual fig orchard with another 415 acres on which figs are grown and 5 acres of roads and farmstead. No other crops are grown. Land is valued at $1,200 per acre.

2. TREES:

The specific variety of fig trees planted in this study is Conadria. The trees are planted at 15 x 20 foot spacing, with 155 trees per acre. Fig trees have a very long production life if they are well maintained. Some fig orchards in the San Joaquin Valley that are still producing a commercial crop are over 75 years old. The life of the orchard at the time of planting is estimated to be 50 years.

3. IRRIGATION:

Pumped water (plus labor) is the irrigation cost. The cost is based on system pumping 24 acre-inches of water 350 feet in a 500-foot well over 500 acres. Water is pumped to the orchard after running through a filtration station into a permanent drip system in the tree rows. The cost of the irrigation system is for the installation of a new pump, well, filtration system, and permanent drip lines. The new irrigation system is installed after the orchard has been laid out and prior to planting. The life of the irrigation system is estimated at 30 years.

Price per acre foot of water will vary by grower in this region depending on power source, cost, various well characteristics, and other irrigation factors. In this study, water is estimated to cost $76.92 per acre foot. No assumption is made about effective rainfall. The amount of water applied to the orchard being established varies each year and is shown in **Table A.**

Table A. Applied Irrigation Water

Year	AcIn/Year
1	4
2	9
3	16
4	18
5+	24

1994 San Joaquin Valley Figs Cost and Return Study (Conadria Variety) UC Cooperative Extension 3

4. ESTABLISHMENT PRACTICES:

Orchard Development: This orchard is established on ground that has not been previously planted in trees or vines. The land is assumed to be slightly rolling and not on a Class I soil. The orchard site is not leveled, thus requiring a drip or sprinkler irrigation system.

Land Preparation: Land preparation begins with a deep ripping, going down five to six feet to break up underlying hardpans which would affect root and water penetration. The ripping is performed by contract operators. Following the ripping, the ground is first disced and then floated by the orchard owner. This breaks up large clods of soil and smooth the ground in advance of planting the trees. All of the operations that prepare the orchard for planting are done in the first year.

Planting: Planting starts by marking the tree location with a stake. Holes are then dug and the trees are planted. The young trees are pruned back soon after planting. Regular pruning and sucker removal begins in the second year and hours and costs required to perform these tasks increase annually. Pruning is performed in the fall months. Removing the suckers is usually performed while weeding crews hand hoe the orchard. In the second year, 10 percent of the trees (16 trees per acre) will have to be replanted.

Orchard Floor Management: Weed control for the orchard begins in the fall with a residual herbicide sprayed along the tree rows. The same chemicals are used for this control during the life of the orchard, but only half of the full rate is used in the first two years; it is increased to the full rate in the third. In spring a contact herbicide is used to control vegetation in the middle of the tree rows with two applications. In the first two seasons, a full rate of the spot spray is used only on 25 percent of the acreage. Beginning in the third year, full rates are again used, but this time on all of the acreage. Discing is also used to control vegetation and is performed four times during the first two years and once per season beginning in year three. Not only is discing used to manage orchard floor vegetation, but it also tills the soil in preparation for being packed, leveled, and smoothed. This operation produces a smooth, hard surface free of debris for efficient mechanical harvesting.

Insect, Disease, and Vertebrate Management: During typical years pest control in fig orchards is limited to controlling rodents, but in exceptionally cool weather a rapid build up of insect pests can occur which may require treatment. Baits are applied through the orchard at bait stations. Arthropod pests are typically not a problem in fig orchards, though serious infestations can occur and may require pest control. No insecticide or disease sprays are assumed to be used for the orchard in this study.

Fertilization:

Nitrogen is the major nutrient required for proper tree growth and optimum fruit yields. Nitrogen fertilizer is spread in a granular form of ammonium nitrate (34-0-0) at increasing rates during orchard establishment and is shown in **Table B.**

Table B. Applied Nitrogen

Year	Pounds Of N/ Acre
1	20
2	40
3	60
4	80
5	100

Establishment Cost

The cost to establish the orchard is used to determine the non-cash overhead expenses, depreciation and interest on investment, for the production years. The establishment cost is the sum of the costs for land preparation, planting, trees, cash overhead and production expenses for growing the trees through the third year. The *Total Accumulated Net Cash Cost* in the third year, shown on **Table 1**, represents the establishment cost. For this study, this cost is $1,955 per acre or $811,325 for the 415 acres of mature orchard is estimated: this cost is shown in **Table 5 (This and subsequent Tables available on UC Davis Cooperative Extension Website).** The establishment cost is spread over the remaining 47 years of the 50 years that the orchard is assumed to be in production.

5. PRODUCTION CULTURAL PRACTICES:

Pruning: Pruning is done by hand in the winter months. Prunings are pushed out of the orchard by a tractor using a brush rake and burned. Suckers are removed by hand crews as they hoe weeds during April.

Fertilization: Nitrogen fertilizer is applied in summer/fall following harvest. Proper levels of nitrogen to be applied to the orchard are determined by leaf analysis. Sampling is usually done in July, before the application of fertilizer. Nitrogen is applied at a rate of 100 pounds of N per acre.

Orchard Floor Management: Weeds in the mature orchard are controlled with chemical and cultural practices as used in the later years of orchard establishment. A combination of residual herbicides is sprayed in a strip along the tree rows to control weeds there throughout the season. Tree row middles are disced once in the spring, to manage resident vegetation on the orchard floor and to prepare the ground to be packed, leveled, and smoothed prior to the first harvest. Vegetation in row middles that are not controlled by cultivation receive two sprays of a contact herbicide during spring and summer.

Insect, Disease and Vertebrate Management: Arthropods and disease pests are commonly not serious enough in a well managed fig orchard to warrant treatment. The only pests that require control in this study are rodents. Commercially available baits are used in bait stations within the orchard in order to manage them during the growing season.

The pesticides and rates mentioned in this cost study are a few of those that are listed in the UC IPM Fig Pest Management Guidelines. Written recommendations are required for most pesticides and are made by licensed pest control advisors. For information and pesticide use permits, contact the local county Agricultural Commissioner's office. For additional information contact the farm advisor in the county of interest.

6. HARVEST:

Harvesting begins in the third year after the orchard is planted. As the yields increase, the cost to harvest also increases until maturity is reached in approximately the tenth year. In this cost study the crop is harvested and sorted by the grower. The number of harvest per year also changes as the orchard matures. In the third year, three harvests are performed. The fourth year requires four harvests, the fifth year figs are harvested five times, and from the sixth year on six harvests are completed annually. In this cost study, the crop is harvested and sorted by the grower.

Fig harvesting begins as the fruit naturally falls to the ground. In the late season crop some figs may cling to the trees, which require growers to use blowers to force those remaining fruit to fall. The sweeper windrows the figs into the middle of the orchard row so that the harvester can pick up the fruit and dump them into field bins. A hand crew may rake the figs that are lying next to the tree out to where a mechanical orchard sweeper can reach them. The figs are hauled from the field to a dry yard. A grower with 500 acres of figs in production is assumed to own his dry yard, and would sort his figs. After sorting, the figs are sold to processors.

For growers that do not own harvesting and packing equipment, the needed equipment for harvesting and packing operations should be removed from the equipment and investment inventories on **Table 5**, and custom harvest and packing charges should be placed in Harvest costs in **Tables 1** and **2**. All of the grower performed harvest and packing costs would be subtracted from Harvest costs in **Tables 1** and **2.**

1994 San Joaquin Valley Figs Cost and Return Study (Conadria Variety) UC Cooperative Extension 5

7. ASSESSMENTS:

Under a state marketing order, mandatory assessment fees are collected by the California Fig Advisory Board (CFAB). These assessments are charged both to the grower and the processor to pay for fig marketing and advertising. Half of the fee of $48 per ton of merchantable fruit (merchantable fruit is destined for dried, or paste markets) is paid by the grower and is shown in this study, while the remaining $24 is paid by the processor. Additionally, a voluntary assessment is also paid by fig growers for research and administration and is managed by the California Fig Institute (CFI). Though the assessment is voluntary it is currently supported by all of the growers. CFI charges growers $5 per ton of merchantable fruit. Both of these assessments are shown as a harvest cost.

8. YIELDS AND RETURNS:

Yields: As noted above, figs most often begin bearing an economic crop in the third year after planting. Typical annual yields for the Conadria variety is measured in pounds for merchantable figs and tons for cull fruit. Typical cull percentages for Conadria figs have ranged between 7-8 percent. This study uses a 7 percent cull rate. The yields shown in **Table C** are from the third year of orchard establishment to maturity.

Table C — **Annual Yield Per Acre**

		Figs – Pounds/Acre		
Year	Tons/Acre	Total	Merchantable	Cull
3	0.20	400	372	28
4	0.80	1,600	1,488	112
5	1.20	2,400	2,232	168
6	1.52	3,040	2,827	213
7	1.80	3,600	3,348	252
8	2.00	4,000	3,720	280
9	2.24	4,480	4,166	314
10+	2.40	4,800	4,464	336

Returns: Conadria figs are used in the paste market. For figs that are sold for paste a price of $0.50 per pound is used. Culled fruit is sold for cattle feed with the grower receiving $0.03 per pound in this study. **Table 7** indicates returns to risk and management at various levels of fig prices and yields. It calculates returns above three levels of cost: operating, cash and total.

9. RISK:

Risk is caused by various sources of uncertainty which include production, price, and financial. Examples of these are insect damage, a decrease in price, and increase in interest rates. The risks associated with fig production should not be underestimated. While this study makes every effort to model a production system based on typical, real world practices, it cannot fully represent financial, agronomic and market risks which affect the profitability and economic viability of fig production. Due to the risk involved, access to a market crucial. A market channel should be determined before any fig orchards are planted and brought into production.

10. LABOR:

Basic hourly wages for workers are $6.00 and $4.51 per hour for machine operators and field workers (irrigator), respectively. Adding 34 percent for Workers Compensation, Social Security, Medicare, insurance and other possible benefits gives the labor rates shown of $8.04 per hour for machine labor and $6.04 per hour for non-machine labor. The labor hours for operations involving machinery are 20 percent higher than the machine hours, to account for extra labor involved in equipment set-up, moving, maintenance, and repair. Wages for managers are not included as a cash cost. Any returns above total costs are considered returns to investment

1994 San Joaquin Valley Figs Cost and Return Study (Conadria Variety) UC Cooperative Extension 6

11. CASH OVERHEAD:

Cash overhead consists of various cash expenses paid out during the year assigned to the whole farm and not to a particular operation. These costs include property taxes, interest on operating capital, office expense, liability and property insurance, sanitation services, leaf analysis, and investment repairs.

Property Tax: Counties charge a base property tax rate of 1 percent on the assessed value of the property. In some counties special assessment districts exist and charge additional taxes on property including equipment, buildings,
and improvements. County taxes are calculated as 1 percent of the average value of the property for this study. Average value equals new cost plus salvage value divided by two on a per acre basis.

Interest On Operating Capital: Interest on operating capital is based on cash operating costs and is calculated monthly until harvest at a nominal rate of 7.89 percent per year. A nominal interest rate is the going market cost of borrowed funds.

Office Expense: Office and business expenses are estimated at $100 per acre. These expenses include office supplies, telephones, bookkeeping, accounting, legal fees, and road maintenance.

Insurance: Insurance for farm investments vary depending on the assets covered and the amount of coverage. Property insurance provides coverage for property loss and is charged at 0.713 percent of the average value of the assets over their useful life. Liability insurance covers accidents on the farm, and costs $615 for the entire farm ($1.23 per acre).

Sanitation Services: Sanitation services provide portable toilets for the orchard and cost the farm $970 annually. The cost for this includes delivery and servicing of toilets.

Leaf Analysis: Analysis for nutrients needed for proper tree growth and fruit development is performed on leaf petiole samples. A cost of $4.50 per acre covers this service. Many fertilization programs are based in part on leaf analysis. Cash overhead costs are found in **Tables 1, 2, 3, 4,** and **5.**

12. NON-CASH OVERHEAD:

Non-cash overhead is comprised of depreciation and interest charged on equipment and other investments. Most of the equipment inventory in typical fig orchards in the San Joaquin Valley is purchased both new and used. This study shows current purchase price for new equipment adjusted to 60 percent of new value to indicate a mix of new and used equipment. Annual equipment and investment costs are shown in **Tables 1, 2,** and **5**. They represent depreciation and opportunity cost for each investment on an annual per acre basis.

Depreciation: Depreciation is a reduction in market value of investments due to wear, obsolescence, and age, and is on a straight line basis. Annual depreciation is calculated as purchase price minus salvage value divided by years the investment is held. The purchase price and years of life are shown in **Table 5**.

Opportunity Costs: Interest is charged on investments to account for income foregone (opportunity cost) that could be received from an alternative investment. The investments are assumed to be owned outright. Therefore, interest on investments is a non-cash cost. Investments include land, orchard, buildings, and equipment. Interest is calculated as the average value of the investment during its useful life, multiplied by 3.72 percent per year. Average value for equipment and buildings equals new cost plus salvage value divided by two on a per acre basis. The average value for land is equal to the purchase price because land does not depreciate. Real interest rates are used on long term assets to show current costs.

13. EQUIPMENT CASH COSTS:

Equipment costs are composed of three parts; non-cash overhead, cash overhead, and operating costs. Both of the overhead factors have been discussed in previous sections. The operating costs consist of fuel, lubrication, and repairs.

In allocating the equipment costs on a per acre basis, the following hourly charges are calculated first and shown in **Table 6.** Repair costs are based on purchase price, annual hours of use, total hours of life, and repair coefficients formulated by the American Society of Agricultural Engineers (ASAE). Fuel and lubrication costs are also determined by ASAE equations based on maximum PTO hp, and type of fuel used. The fuel and repair cost per acre for each operation in **Table 2** is determined by multiplying the total hourly operating cost in **Table 6** for each piece of equipment used for the cultural practice by the number of hours per acre for that operation. Tractor time is 10 percent higher than implement time for a given operation to account for setup time. Prices for on-farm delivery of diesel and gasoline are $0.85 and $1.17 per gallon, respectively.

14. ACKNOWLEDGMENT:

Appreciation is expressed to the California Fig Advisory Board, California Fig Institute, and the fig growers in the San Joaquin Valley who participated in this study. Their information and expertise, so generously provided, helped make the production of this study possible.

Calimyrna Figs to Market

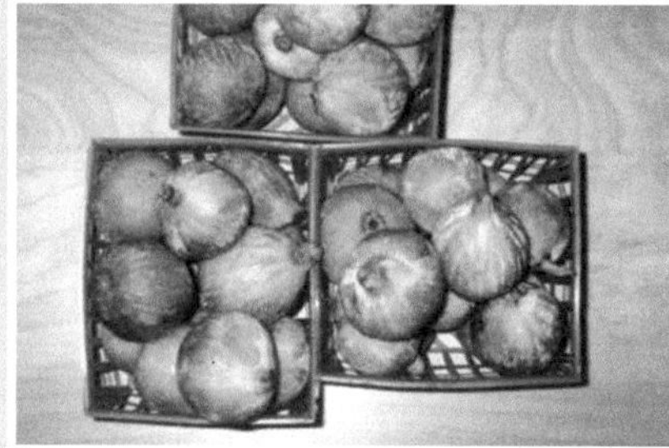

Calimyrna Figs at Home

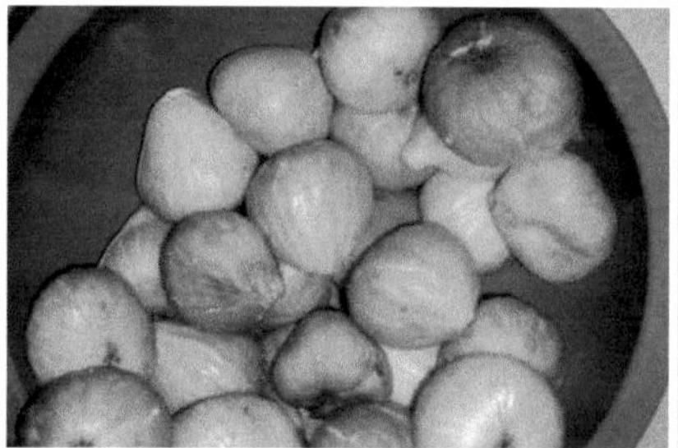

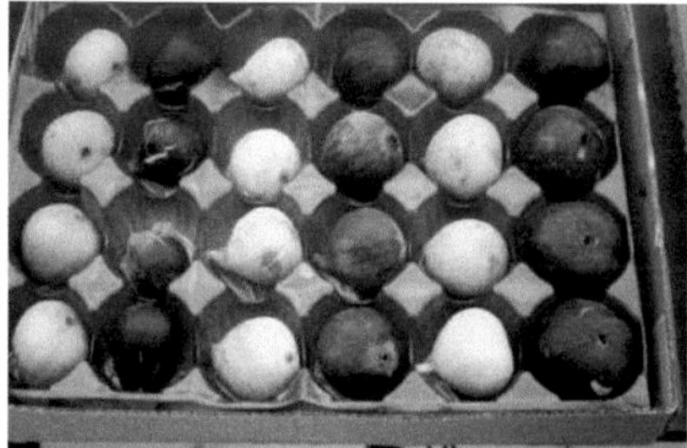

Calimyrna and Mission Figs in California

1994 San Joaquin Valley Figs Cost and Return Study (Conadria Variety) UC Cooperative Extension 8

Chapter Three

FROM ORCHARD TO BANQUET TABLE

Figs are an excellent staple for the health food counter at restaurants, farmers markets, and the gourmet banquet table. Use figs in your recipes, whether you run a small catering operation, a roadside dessert stop, a beach food cart, a stand in your local mall, or an urban gourmet dining room.

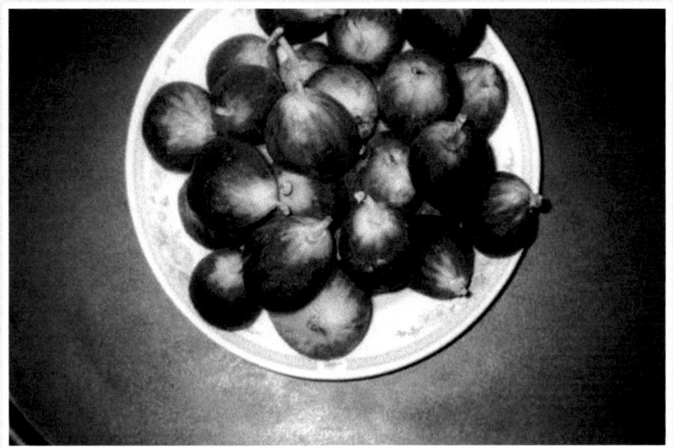

Healthy Honey Figs

PREPARATION

Add figs to food that need a touch of sweetness. If your only experience with figs comes from eating Fig Newtons, dealing with the squat, bulbous, and thoroughly wrinkled whole fruit can be a bit confusing. Figs, both fresh and dried, are easy to handle.

Some people peel the skin back from the stem end to expose the flesh. The more fastidious chef holds the fruit by the stem end, cuts the fruit into quarters from the apex, spreads the section apart, lifts the flesh from the skin with a knife blade, and discards the stem and skin. Commercially, figs are peeled by immersion for one minute in boiling lye water or a boiling solution of sodium bicarbonate. In warm, humid climate figs are generally eaten fresh and raw without peeling and they are often served with cream and sugar. Peeled or unpeeled, figs may be stewed or cooked in various ways (pies, pudding, cakes, bread, other bakery products), added to ice cream mixes, jam, marmalade, paste and compotes. They are sometimes commercially can-dried.

Shopping Guidelines

Figs, whether fresh or dried, should be firm, but still yield slightly to the touch. If dried figs are rock hard, do not buy them. If fresh figs seem mushy, they are too ripe and will not deliver full flavor.

Healthy figs and ripe mission figs will always have a rich color. Look for shapely, plump figs with unbruised, unbroken skins and a mild fragrance (sour smelling figs indicate spoilage). Figs should be just soft to the touch, but not mushy.

Fresh figs deteriorate rapidly, usually within a few days. They will stay fresh for about three days when stored in the refrigerator. Dried figs, by contrast, will keep for months when stored in an airtight bag in the refrigerator.

Because figs are extremely sticky, they can be difficult to eat. Chilling the figs for an hour before cutting will help prevent them from sticking to your equipment. The flavor and fragrance of fresh figs are best, however, at room temperature. Simply quarter the figs lengthwise and place them on a plate. A sprinkle of orange or lemon juice will heighten their flavor.

Figs also work well with walnuts or almonds. Use dried figs in recipes that can replace apricots, dates, or other fruit. Try them in whole-wheat muffins, cookies and cake fillings. Chopping dried figs provides an interesting texture to fresh fruit salads; combine them with bananas or berries. For a special vegetable side dish, sprinkle chopped dried figs over baked sweet potatoes or winter squash, or stir the figs into mashed sweet potatoes or in squash. Thread skewers with fresh or dried figs and grill with kebabs, or offer them on their own as a barbecue dessert.

The following recipes are for high-yield quantities and will work well in your catering, food stall or restaurant dishes:

Fruit Croissants - Yields 12 ½ dozen (1½ oz) croissants

3½ oz yeast
4 lbs water
5 oz nonfat dry milk
14 oz granulated sugar
Mix water, yeast, dry milk and sugar on low speed for 1 minute.

2½ oz salt
7 oz whole eggs
5 oz butter, melted
Add salt, eggs and butter. Mix on low speed for 4 minutes.

4 lbs, 4 oz flour, unbleached bread
2 lbs 6 oz flour, high gluten

Add flours. Mix on low speed for 4 minutes. Allow to triple in size in bowl. Punch down. Scale into 14 oz pieces.

6 lbs butter

Sheet each piece into 18" x 54" rectangle. Spot 36" with butter. Do 3-three-folds with a minimum of 30 minutes rest in refrigerator between each fold. Refrigerate dough 8 to 12 hours.

4 lbs 10 oz fig filling (below)

Do a final three-fold and sheet 3/8" thick. Cut into croissants. Spoon fig filling across wide end. Roll up and shape into croissants. Spray with egg wash and top with streusel (below), if desired. Bake at 350° F for 15 minutes.

Fig Filling

2 lbs 4 oz California fig paste or California diced figs
1 lb 8 oz water
1 lb 5 oz granulated sugar
2 oz vanilla

Combine fig paste or diced figs, water and sugar in kettle. Heat to boiling and simmer 10 to 20 minutes. Turn into food processor or mixer bowl and process or beat on high until smooth. Stir in vanilla. Add water, as needed, and mix until desired consistency for spreading.

Streusel

8 oz butter
12 oz granulated sugar
12 oz flour

Combine all ingredients and mix until crumbly.

Chunky Fig Bread - Yields 19 loaves (16 oz loaves)

12 oz yeast
5 lbs 14 oz water

Dissolve yeast in water. Set aside.
10 lbs bread flour
1 lb granulated sugar
3 oz salt
1 lb butter
2 oz lemon juice
9 oz nonfat dry milk

Combine flour, sugar, salt, butter, lemon juice and nonfat dry milk in mixer bowl. Add yeast mixture. Mix on low speed for 1 minute, then on high until dough cleans bowl. Mix 2 minutes longer. Final dough temperature, 80° F. Scale dough into 16 oz pieces.

Flatten each piece and spread with 2 oz fig filling (below). Roll up as a jelly roll. Seal seam and ends. Pan. Brush top with egg wash and sprinkle with streusel (below). Proof for 45 minutes at 100° F dry or 95° F wet (cold wet). Bake at 350° F for 35 to 40 minutes.

Fig Filling

9 oz California fig paste or California diced figs
12½ oz water
10½ oz granulated sugar
2¼ oz lemon juice concentrate

Combine fig paste or diced figs, water and sugar in kettle. Heat to boiling and simmer 10 to 20 minutes. Turn into food processor or mixer bowl and process or beat on high until smooth. Stir in lemon juice concentrate. Add water, as needed, and mix until desired consistency for spreading.

Streusel (See above recipe)

Fig Danish - Yields 14 dozen (4 oz each)

1 lb yeast
8 lbs 5 oz water

Combine yeast and part of water. Set aside.

2 lbs 8 oz butter
2 lbs 8 oz granulated sugar
5 oz salt
½ oz ground nutmeg
3 lbs whole eggs
12 oz nonfat dry milk
2 oz vanilla

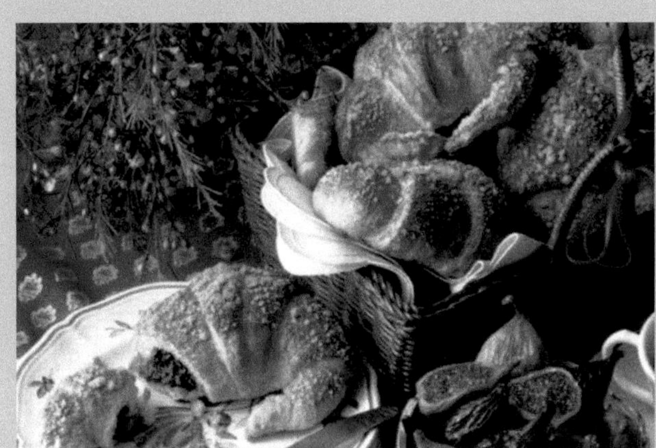

Fig Croissants

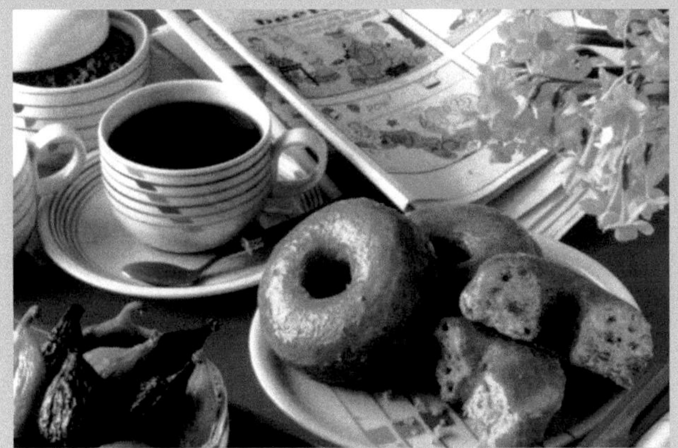

Fig Doughnut

Mix butter, sugar, salt, and nutmeg together. Beat in eggs, nonfat dry milk and vanilla.

16 lbs 10 oz bread flour

Add dissolved yeast and remaining water alternately with flour. Mix only until smooth. ***Do not over mix.***

6 lbs butter

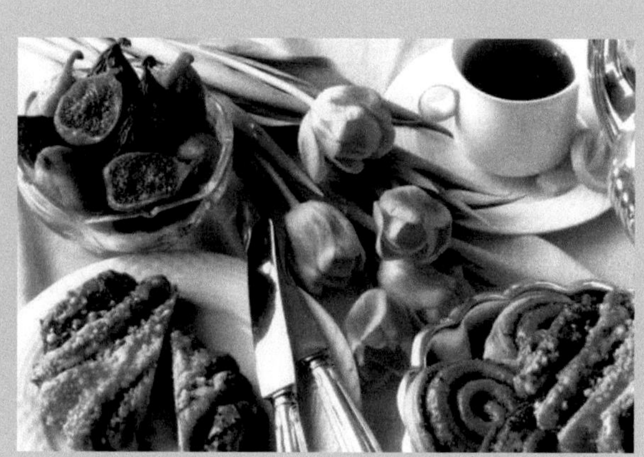

Fig Danish

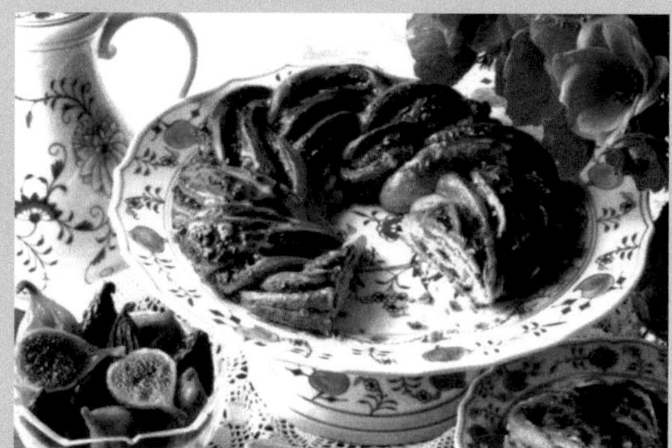

Fig Coffercake

Let dough rest for 20 minutes. Sheet dough for a three-fold and spread butter over 2/3 of dough. Give dough three folds with a 90° turn each time and a 20-minute rest in cooler (40° F) between folds. Rest dough 30 minutes after last fold.

Sheet dough to 16" wide and ½" thick. Spread with fig filling (below). Shape as desired. Place on parchment-lined pan. Brush with egg wash and sprinkle with streusel, if desired. Proof in cool wet box (100° F). Bake at 350° F for 13 to 15 minutes.

Fig Filling

7 lbs California fig paste or California diced figs
4 lbs 14 oz water
4 lbs 2 oz granulated sugar
6 oz vanilla

Combine fig paste or diced figs, water and sugar in kettle. Heat to boiling and simmer 10 to 20 minutes. Turn into food processor or mixer bowl and process or beat on high until smooth. Stir in vanilla. Add water, as needed, and mix until desired consistency for spreading.

Streusel

2 lbs butter
3 lbs granulated sugar
3 lbs flour

Combine all ingredients and mix until crumbly.

Fruit Doughnuts - Yields 7½ dozen (1½ oz each)

5 oz yeast
2 lbs water

Crumble yeast and dissolve in part of the water. Set aside.

4 lbs 2 oz bread flour
1½ oz baking powder
4 oz nonfat dry milk
1 oz salt
10 oz shortening
10 oz fig filling (below)
8 oz eggs, whole

Combine remaining ingredients in mixer bowl. Add yeast mixture and remaining water. Mix 1 minute on low; then on high until dough has formed a ball and cleaned the bowl. Continue mixing 2 minutes more. Rest 30 minutes; punch down. Rest 30 minutes longer and punch down again. Sheet ½" to ¾" thick. Cut into doughnuts. Proof at 100° F to 95° F wet until more than double in bulk. Fry at 360° F until golden brown.

Fig Filling

4½ oz California fig paste or California diced figs
3 oz water
2½ oz granulated sugar
¼ oz vanilla

Combine fig paste or diced figs, water and sugar in kettle. Heat to boiling and simmer 10 to 20 minutes. Turn into food processor or mixer bowl and process or beat on high until smooth. Stir in vanilla. Add water, as needed, and mix until desired consistency.

Fig Coffee Cake - Yields 20 cakes (12 oz each)

7 oz yeast
15 oz water or milk

Dissolve yeast in water. Set aside.

17 oz granulated sugar
1½ oz salt
1 lb 5 oz butter

Cream sugar, salt and butter together.

10½ oz whole eggs
½ oz grated lemon peel

Add eggs and lemon peel; mix well.

2 lbs 11 oz water or milk

Add water and 2/3 of the flour and mix well. Stir in yeast mixture.

7 lbs 7 oz bread flour

Add remaining flour and mix until dough is smooth with no lumps. Allow dough to rise 2 hours. Punch down. Scale dough into 12 oz pieces. Sheet each piece to 6"x12".

Fig Filling (below)

Spread each sheet with 4 oz fig filling. Roll into tube. Shape into circle and seal ends together. Alternate cuts on top. Brush with egg wash and sprinkle with streusel (below). Proof 45 minutes at 100° F dry or 95° F wet. Bake at 350° F for 30 to 34 minutes.

2 lbs 4 oz California fig paste or California diced figs
1 lb 8 oz water
1 lb 5 oz granulated sugar
4½ oz lemon juice concentrate

Combine fig paste or diced figs, water and sugar in kettle. Heat to boiling and simmer 10 to 20 minutes. Turn into food processor or mixer bowl and process or beat on high until smooth. Stir in lemon juice concentrate. Add water, as needed, and mix until desired consistency for spreading.

Streusel

4 oz butter
6 oz granulated sugar
6 oz flour

Combine all ingredients and mix until crumbly.

Printed in the United States
by Baker & Taylor Publisher Services